The Fasting Handbook

Dining from an Empty Bowl

Jeremy Safron

Celestial Arts
Berkeley | Toronto

Celestial Arts
P.O. Box 7123
Berkeley, California 94707
www.tenspeed.com

Distributed in Australia by Simon and Schuster Australia, in Canada by Ten Speed Press Canada, in New Zealand by Southern Publishers Group, in South Africa by Real Books, and in the United Kingdom and Europe by Airlift Book Company.

Disclaimer: This book is designed to provide information. It is every individual's responsibility to make his own decisions. By having all the necessary information, you can make better choices. This book does not heal people. People heal themselves. As with all things in life, think before you act. Make wise choices based on education and experience. Always diagnose and get many opinions on any area. The carpenter's adage of measure twice and cut once always applies. Take your time and use wisdom and discernment in all situations. Loving Foods and Jeremy Safron make no promises. We believe in promising nothing and delivering big. Health and healing are your own unique process with yourself. Each individual is different, and so each solution is different. To heal yourself, know yourself first. Make use of the information in this book to empower yourself and others and be your most divine and powerful self.

Cover and Interior Design by Leslie Waltzer, Crowfoot Design

Library of Congress Cataloging-in-Publication Data is on file with the publisher

First printing, 2005

Printed in the U.S.A.

1 2 3 4 5 6 7 8 9 10 — 09 08 07 06 05

Dedication

This book is dedicated to all the animals and plants who know
the secret of self-healing, and to Mother Maui.

Acknowledgments

I would like to acknowledge and thank Herbert Shelton, T. C. Fry,
The Natural Hygiene Movement, Annie Jubb, Victoria Bidwell, Sena Miller,
Gabriel Cousins, Jah Rastafari, the Native American Church, the Essenes,
my Mom, Senia Feiner, Enchantments in New York City, Angelica's Herbs
in New York City, Dr. Ann Wigmore, and Victoras Kulvinskas.

Most of all, I'd like to thank Jai from New Jersey for handing me the book
Survival into the 21st Century and for all the shots of wheatgrass.

Contents

Introduction

Types of Fasts and Fasting Ceremonies

Fasting On

Fasting From

Practices for Cleansing

Practices for Cleansing *(continued)*

Custom-Tailored Fasts

Fasting Assistants

Self-Empowerment Questionnaire

Recommended Reading

Glossary

Raw Truth Catalog

Introduction

What Is Fasting?

Fasting allows our body to heal itself. It is the practice of cleansing through the consumption of specific substances. By putting less in, we are able to focus on healing and being, rather than eating and doing. Ingesting only pure food or water of a certain type allows the body to heal and recover faster. A massive amount of daily energy goes to processing the things we consume. When we choose to eat very simply, the body can go to work removing obstacles and clearing toxic debris.

There are actually only two types of disease—assimilation or elimination. That is to say, you are either getting less of what you need or you are holding on to unwanted material that must be removed. Certain fasting practices allow your body the opportunity to remove harmful toxic substances, while others help you obtain the necessary components to heal, rejuvenate, and function in an optimal way.

The concept of "less is best" is the faster's adage. When we do not use parts of our body, those parts are given a better opportunity to heal. Although in some beliefs fasting is the consumption of nothing at all, any abstention or austerity can be a form of fasting. Fasting brings us closer to ourselves and offers us the opportunity to press the reset button on our body and life. By fasting, we can create new beginnings. A fast is an opportunity to come into greater self-knowledge and self-discipline. By fasting, we get to know ourselves in new ways and define our future. Fasting is a time of rejuvenation and rebirth. Life is renewed and health is restored by bringing the body and its organs back into ideal functioning.

One may not reach the dawn save by the path of night.
— *THE PROPHET,* KHALIL GIBRAN

Why Fast?

People fast for a variety of reasons—primarily for physical health, spiritual practice, emotional expression, and brain power. Because of the pollutants in the Western world, much of the air and food is poisoned, and many commercially corrupted people have consumed the edible media of today's society. Toxins brought into the body are stored there and may lie dormant and cause cancer and other degenerative diseases. To help the body extend its life and function more optimally, these toxins must be removed.

Many religious holidays and spiritual practices require fasting as a part of the ceremony. Spiritual leaders around the world fast to become empty so they can be filled with the spirit of god. Some fasts are lengthy, while others are short. Some examples include:

Yom Kippur is the Hebrew holiday of cleansing, where no food or drink is consumed for twenty-four hours while people atone for their sins. Pieces of bread, as a representation of sins, are cast out into flowing water to be cast out of the body and soul.

Ramadan is an Islamic holiday where only water is consumed from sunrise until sundown for thirty days.

Lent is a Christian holy time where a certain type of food is given up for six weeks to help atone for sin and to share in the events that occurred before the Resurrection.

In preparation for Native American sweat lodges, participants fast to get ready for this purification ritual.

People who find themselves in emotionally exaggerated situations choose not to eat food because so much of their energy is focused on the challenge at hand. On the other hand, when people are happy, they require less food.

Fasting can also help the mind maintain focus. By not spending extra energy to digest food, that energy can be added to our brain power to help us stay clear for such things as exams, public speaking, important meetings, or crucial events.

Planning a Fast

To properly heal and cleanse our body, it is important to properly plan a fast. Planning for a fast can be relatively simple or highly complex depending on the type and length of the fast. The first thing to do is decide what kind of fast you want to experience and how long you will remain on this fast.

Once you decide on a fast, it is important to make certain that you have all the items you need to follow the fast to completion. If you are planning to do some of the more intense fasts, make sure someone knows about it and is able to assist you if needed. For some fasts, it is important to have free time to process and cleanse, so if you choose a more rapid practice, it is beneficial to have only one obligation, healing.

Some of the fasts in this book allow you to continue with your daily life, while others require that you be at home relaxing. It is important to choose a fast that complements your current lifestyle. You will find that when healing is needed, the opportunity presents itself. If you are planning any organ cleanses or wish to gain the assistance of healers (for example, massage or colonic), be sure to schedule these in advance.

It is often beneficial to begin a fast with the new moon. The new moon is a symbol of beginnings and change. If you are creating a fourteen-day fast, it's nice to start with the new moon and to begin to eat (breakfast) on the full moon.

A fast is a time of purification. Choose to take space on your own to reflect within and gain innerstanding.

Starting and Ending a Fast

The opening and closing of a fast are crucial to how the body rejuvenates and recovers. It is very important to be gentle with your body. A good rule of thumb is to take twice as long coming out of a fast as going into one. When you begin to fast, it is often helpful to lessen the intake of food at meals and to spread your meals farther apart (possibly even cut back to one major meal a day). It is also helpful to eat food that contains a high water content. Food containing a high water content will help your body become more ready to begin your cleanse.

When concluding a fast, it is important to begin to reintroduce the proper digestive bacteria and to get your digestion flowing again. Juices and fruits are great fast breakers, and then you can move to sprouted and cultured foods to bring the digestive bacteria back in line and renew metabolic processes.

Patience is a virtue, and when we move into a cleansing process, our mind becomes resistant and attempts to reengage a pattern of imbalance. It can take a great amount of will power to begin a fast and even more to continue it, but it is ending a fast that is most challenging. It is crucial to break a fast in a slow and even way. Take your time and adjust to eating again. Many a great fast is ended incorrectly by jumping right back into food because of desire or outside influences. The breaking of a fast is sacred and, if done correctly, allows our body to heal and develop in powerful new ways.

If a fast is broken incorrectly, it can actually concentrate toxins in the body and cause further ailments. It is important to be realistic and only set goals for a fast that you know you can achieve. Start small and do a few one- to three-day fasts before beginning a lengthy fast. Be prepared and plan your fast well, and it will be a joyful and rejuvenating experience.

Length of a Fast

The length of a fast is always based on an individual's situation. The cleaner our body, the longer we can fast, and the easier it will be to fast. The question of how you know when to break your fast is very personal. When first fasting, it is best to create a fasting program that you know to be within your potential to complete. Once you have experimented with different fasts and cleanses, you can go as long as possible, or until your body has cleaned out.

One way to know that the body is clean is that a very sweet taste begins to appear in the mouth and your sweat smells very fragrant. Another great method for knowing the body is clean is that real hunger begins to surface. Real hunger is your interest in taking in nourishment through food, as opposed to false hunger, which is based on cravings due to addiction.

Long-term fasting is often used to clear away old patterns and to free the body of toxins. Some experts believe that as long as it took you to get where you are, it will take equally as long to get back. This means that, if you ate toxic foods for twenty years, it will take twenty years of eating good food for your body to naturally detoxify. Fasting gives you the ability to remove toxins at a far more rapid rate. Some of the fasts in this book remove toxins at a rate of two to one, while others are more like one hundred to one (one hundred days of toxic intake removed in one day).

Lengthy fasts can truly bring our body back to a healthy set point. From there, we can build our body into our ideal self.

Maintenance fasting is the practice of fasting for short periods of time, such as one day a week, once a month, or on the full moon. This type of fasting is used to give the body a rest and the opportunity to rejuvenate, whereas lengthy fasts put the body into rapid detox. Maintenance fasts are very useful once you have cleansed your body and help keep you functioning at an optimal level.

Short-term fasts are often used to gain focus and spiritual power or to give us the opportunity to experience ourselves. During the first day of a cleanse, you are often still processing the previous day's consumptions. Short fasts can give your body the chance to catch up and get back to empty before you start eating again.

There is great power to be gained by fasting; use it wisely.

Mental and Emotional Detoxification

There are many reasons why toxins and other harmful substances stay in the body. When toxic minerals or chemicals enter your system, your body often cannot deal with processing them all at once. Your body will remove what it can and store the rest away to be dealt with at a future date. Many people who live a toxic lifestyle do not give their body an opportunity to process out this old waste. Eventually, this waste builds up until the person dies of internal poisoning or the body creates a tumor or growth.

Extreme emotion can also store toxins in the body. Even the small amount of airborne toxins or toxic household items may be locked into the body by emotion. Sometimes when under stress, people consume toxic foods (junk food, meat, synthetic food). Often emotions act like glue, keeping this toxic material in the body. When fasting and cleansing, it is necessary to release these emotions. Some people fast, and, when their emotions surface, they start eating or don't deal with their emotions and are unable to release the toxic material stored in the body. Sometimes self-reassurance or affirmations can help in releasing and rebuilding our body. It is very important to go through the emotional detox when fasting. Thoughts, memories, and feelings that come up want to be processed and dealt with. It may be challenging, yet on the other side of the resurfacing issue is a healing on every level. When the feeling is recognized and transformed, it allows a great amount of toxic matter stored in the body to be released and purified out of the body. Many toxic thoughts and visual and auditory stimuli can also cause poisons around us to get stored away in the body. Cleaning up our language and making healthy choices about what we want to expose ourselves to can lead to great cleansing. By making changes in our inner self, we change what our body is made of. You are what you eat, and you are also what you think and feel.

Fasting with a Partner

It can often be helpful to have a fasting partner. This person can inspire you to be strong in times of cleansing and can be a companion to share juice or prana or whatever you might be fasting on. Fasting together is a wonderful way to bond with your mate. Fasting as a family can bring greater community to the home. Fasting partners are a bountiful source of moral support. While fasting, it is important to go through emotional cleansing. Having someone there to talk to and process with is very strengthening.

Fasting Alone

When fasting alone, it is a good idea to tell someone you are going on a fast (a friend, spouse, or family member). This person can help give you support by asking you how the fast is going and will often be inspired to fast as well (and then you have a fasting partner). By letting someone know you are fasting, you can call on him or her if you need something (like more oranges or an enema bag). This is especially helpful if you are taking quiet time while fasting and don't wish to go to town. Letting someone know you are fasting also helps hold space for your successful cleanse.

Fasticians

A fasting counselor or fastician is someone who can coach you through your fast. This person will monitor your progress and often suggest a specific program or series of cleanses to assist you in obtaining optimal health. When cleansing, a well-experienced opinion can be a fabulous guide on the path of healing.

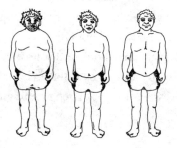

Types of Fasts and Fasting Ceremonies

The following is a collection of various fasting techniques. As with all things, use common sense and remember that it is a sign of wisdom to ask questions of those with a larger range of experience. In this part of the book, you will find explanations of certain fasts, as well as recipes and a day-by-day fasting schedule. These techniques lead you into and out of the actual fast. The "Fasting On" section contains fasts in which only certain foods are consumed. The "Fasting From" section is an austerity guide that you can use to remove items from daily intake. Feel free to use these fasts as a starting point to create your own custom-tailored fast.

Fasting On

Air

Air or dry fasting is the consumption of no food or water whatsoever for a specified period of time. Dry fasting is often done for short periods of time. Animals in the wild when recovering from injury or in later stages of disease will dry fast. This is sometimes due to the fact that the animal cannot get to a food or water source or all the animal's energy is required for healing. We can survive for months without food, for days without water, yet only minutes without air. Air contains prana or chi, a universal energy source that can nourish a body. Many great yogis can survive purely on prana. When we are in dire need of cleansing and healing, it can be of great benefit to minimize consumption. This gives the body the opportunity to truly heal and recover. Air fasts are probably the most intense and are only recommended for the experienced faster. Be certain that you have a fasting coach or partner for this type of fast.

Dry Fast

	Breakfast	Lunch	Dinner
Day 1 in	Fruit	Smoothie	Juice
Day 2 in	Juice	Juice	Juice
Day 3 in	Consume as much water as possible before beginning dry fast.		
Day 4	Consume only air and breathe deeply. Continue for only one day.		
Day 1 out	Water (sip slowly)	Juice	Juice
Day 2 out	Juice	Juice	Juice
Day 3 out	Juice	Smoothie	Smoothie
Day 4 out	Juice	Smoothie	Fruit
Day 5 out	Begin to return to a balanced diet including sprouts and fermented foods.		

Water

Water fasting is the process of consuming only water. When you water-fast, you are flushing out the toxins stored in the body. Water fasting is the quickest way to cleanse and purify the system. Since you will be constantly flowing water through the body to carry away toxins, it is extremely helpful to do a kidney cleanse before beginning a water fast. It is very important when you are water fasting to have a good source of water. The best water sources are reverse osmosis, charged water, and distilled water. The more alkaline the water, the greater the healing benefits. You can create alkaline water (7 pH and above) by following the recipe that follows. Water fasting is a traditional fast, since many people consider water to be the ultimate healer. Your body is more than 80 percent water, and by consuming large amounts of pure water, your body has the ability to rejuvenate faster. It is ideal to consume as much water as possible to get the greatest benefits.

Charged Water

1 glass gallon jar
1 gallon distilled (water with no minerals)
1 quartz crystal (well formed and naturally grown)
7 fresh-cut blades of wheatgrass
3 teaspoons seawater or one pinch sea salt

Place all ingredients in the glass jar. Leave the jar out in the sun for at least one day. (Full moon–charged water is great too!) Your water is now charged.

Water Fast

	Breakfast	*Lunch*	*Dinner*
Day 1 in	Fruit	Smoothie	Juice
Day 2 in	Juice	Juice	Juice
Day 3 in	Water	Water	Water
Day 4	Continue on only water for as long as desired.		
Day 1 out	Juice	Juice	Juice
Day 2 out	Juice	Juice	Juice
Day 3 out	Juice	Smoothie	Smoothie
Day 4 out	Juice	Smoothie	Fruit
Day 5 out	Fruit	Fruit	Fruit
Day 6 out	Begin to return to a balanced diet including sprouts and fermented foods.		

Coconut Water

The water from the nut of the coconut palm is almost identical to human blood plasma (which makes up 55 percent of our blood). Coconut water is naturally filtered by a tree for more than nine months and is sealed sterile inside of the shell. Coco water fasting is easier on the body than pure water fasting because of the rich organic minerals and micronutrients contained within. Therefore, the body can go far longer on coco water than on distilled water. Coconut water is one of the highest natural sources of electrolytes and allows the body to maintain a balance of energy and exist in an alkaline environment.

Coconut Water Fast

	Breakfast	Lunch	Dinner
Day 1 in	Fruit	Smoothie	Juice
Day 2 in	Juice	Juice	Juice
Day 3	Consume as much coconut water as possible for as long as you choose.		
Day 1 out	Juice	Juice	Juice
Day 2 out	Juice	Smoothie	Smoothie
Day 3 out	Juice	Smoothie	Fruit
Day 4 out	Begin to return to a balanced diet including sprouts and fermented foods.		

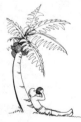

Grass

Grass fasting is the consumption of only chlorophyll-rich grasses. Grasses such as wheat, corn, rye, and oat all provide a wealth of nutrition as well as a high concentration of chlorophyll. Grass fasts are great for removing toxins from the intestinal wall and breaking up old mucoid matter. Grass fasts can also help build the body. Wheatgrass, for example, can provide all the necessary nutrition to the body and is considered a whole food or superfood. All amino acids and basic proteins are contained within grasses. Grasses are also great for colonic implants. Fasting on grass can cause the body to detoxify at a more rapid rate. When undergoing a grass fast, dizziness and nausea often accompany the cleanse because of the amount of toxins released.

Grass Fast

	Breakfast	Lunch	Dinner
Day 1 in	Fruit	Blender soup	Juice
Day 2 in	Grass	Juice	Juice
Day 3 in	Grass	Grass	Grass
Day 4	Continue on only grass for as long as desired.		
Day 1 out	Grass	Juice	Juice
Day 2 out	Grass	Juice	Juice
Day 3 out	Grass	Juice	Blender soup
Day 4 out	Grass	Smoothie	Soup
Day 5 out	Grass	Smoothie	Salad
Day 6 out	Begin to return to a balanced diet including sprouts and fermented foods.		

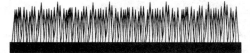

Lemonade or Master Cleanser

Fasting using lemonade is highly beneficial because of the enormously high alkalinity of lemons. Master Cleanser is a variation of lemonade that adds spice to induce internal cleansing and works as a vasodilator (opening veins and arteries). Both cleansers are effective.

Master Cleanser

1/2 cup lemon juice
1/4 teaspoon cayenne powder
Honey, dates, or maple syrup for sweetening

Place all ingredients in a one-gallon glass jar and shake. Sweeten to taste with honey, dates, or maple syrup.

Makes 1 gallon.

Electrolyte Lemonade

1 gallon charged water
1/2 cup lemon juice
1/4 teaspoon sea salt
1/8 teaspoon vanilla
1/4 teaspoon flax oil (butterscotch)
Honey, dates, or maple syrup for sweetening

Place all ingredients in a gallon glass jar and shake well. Sweeten to taste with honey, dates, or maple syrup.

Makes 1 gallon

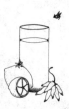

Lemonade or Master Cleanser Fast

	Breakfast	*Lunch*	*Dinner*
Day 1 in	Fruit	Blender soup	Juice
Day 2 in	Juice	Juice	Juice
Day 3	Consume as much lemonade or master cleanser as desired for as long as you choose.		
Day 1 out	Lemonade	Juice	Juice
Day 2 out	Juice	Juice	Juice
Day 3 out	Juice	Smoothie	Blender soup
Day 4 out	Juice	Blender soup	Salad
Day 5 out	Begin to return to a balanced diet including sprouts and fermented foods.		

Juice

Juice fasting is one of the more traditional long-term fasts. Juice fasting is the consumption of only juice. Juice provides a wide range of nutrients to help sustain the body during periods of abstinence from food. Through juice fasting, it is possible to live your daily life and still be on a cleanse. It is important to be certain that you can get as much juice as you want. Juice fasting can only be done with fresh juices. Packaged or bottled juices often are pasteurized (no enzymes). It is important to use only organic juices. The juice of a sprayed or chemically fertilized vegetable can have five times as many toxins as its whole unjuiced counterpart.

Juice fasting is highly beneficial for cleansing the cells. Juice is essentially organic water distilled by a plant with organic vitamins, cell salts, and minerals concentrated in it. Organic water is plant processed and filtered rather than machine filtered. Plants spend many months filtering the water that becomes stored in their leaves, stems, roots, and fruits. By providing clean water, the cells can easily release toxins and cleanse any unwanted substances from the body. Some juice fasts are done on only one type of juice (usually short term), while some are done on combinations. Traditional juice fasts are done for 7, 14, 30, 60, 90, and even 120 days. Juice will oxidize very quickly if made in a centrifugal juicer and must be consumed immediately. Juicing in a masticating or tricherating juicer will oxidize in about two to eight hours, and pressed juice will last as long as twenty-four hours before losing most of its value. The more vital the juice, the more nourishment it can provide the body. Fresh juice is rejuvenating and detoxifying on a cellular level and is a powerful way to heal and renew the body.

Mono Juice Fast

	Breakfast	*Lunch*	*Dinner*
Day 1 in	Fruit	Blender soup	Juice
Day 2 in	Juice	Blender soup	Juice
Day 3	Choose one type of juice and continue for as long as you choose.		
Day 1 out	Juice	Juice	Juice
Day 2 out	Juice	Juice	Blender soup
Day 3 out	Juice	Juice	Blender soup
Day 4 out	Juice	Smoothie	Soup
Day 5 out	Juice	Smoothie	Salad
Day 6 out	Begin to return to a balanced diet including sprouts and fermented foods.		

Multijuice Fast

	Breakfast	Lunch	Dinner
Day 1 in	Fruit	Blender soup	Juice
Day 2 in	Juice	Blender soup	Juice
Day 3	Choose from the list of combinations and continue for as long as you choose. As a general guideline, it is helpful to use fruit juices in the morning, vegetable juices in the afternoon, and return to fruit juices in the evening. If working with sugar imbalances, kidney disorders, or yeast/candida, focus mostly on nonsweet or starchy fruit and vegetable juices.		
Day 1 out	Juice	Juice	Juice
Day 2 out	Juice	Juice	Blender soup
Day 3 out	Juice	Juice	Blender soup
Day 4 out	Juice	Smoothie	Soup
Day 5 out	Juice	Smoothie	Salad
Day 6 out	Begin to return to a balanced diet including sprouts and fermented foods.		

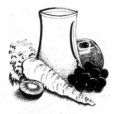

Jeremy's Favorite Juices and Combos

WATERMELON

Watermelons have the highest content of cellular-contained water of any fruit. This makes them ideal for fasting and cleansing. Watermelon juice is very refreshing, and its high water content helps remove toxic debris on a cellular level. Watermelon can be juiced with the rind for chlorophyll and to help cleanse the liver. Melon juice is best done separately from other juices because of the rapid rate of absorption into the body through the stomach lining. If possible, press or blend your watermelon juice to maintain integrity and reduce oxidation.

PANINI

Panini, also known as the prickly pear, is the fruit of a cactus. This fruit has similar benefits to aloe vera. The fruit comes in green and purple and is extremely sweet. It has many small seeds and juices quite well in a Champion juicer or a juice press. The panini is covered in many tiny, thorny spines, so be very careful when handling it. It is best to peel it before juicing. Cut off the top and bottom and then slice a line down one end and peel back the skin. Put the fruit through the juicer and enjoy.

GREEN PAPAYA

Green papaya contains a plethora of enzymes. This fruit is so enzymatically active that it can digest itself and many other foods including old material (especially proteins). Papaya seeds themselves are a vermifuge, an agent that causes the expulsion of worms and parasites from the body. To juice the green papaya, cut off the top where the stem is and then cut it lengthwise in half. Scoop out the seeds and save some for blending. Cut the papaya into strips for juicing or into chunks for blending. The papaya can be juiced with or without the skin. Although the skin is bitter, it has many healing benefits such as tannins (antioxidants)and extra high enzyme activity. Use caution when ingesting papaya skin, as the enzymes can actually burn your tongue.

Sweet Grass

PINEAPPLE AND WHEATGRASS

Pineapples are extremely high in bromelain, a crucial enzyme in the breaking down of foods. Bromelain can help digest food and can often settle the stomach. Wheatgrass, one of nature's simplest medicines, is a great source of chlorophyll and other vital minerals. The combination of the two is less detoxifying than straight wheatgrass but has a great taste. Combine 15 ounces of pineapple juice with one ounce of wheatgrass juice. Stir and enjoy.

Volcano Blood Builder

COCONUT · WHEATGRASS · BEET

Coconut water is almost identical in composition to human blood plasma. You can drink it, or it can be used intravenously (plasma makes up 55 percent of our blood). Wheatgrass juice is one of the highest sources of chlorophyll. Human hemin (the source of hemoglobin, the oxygen carrier) is very similar to chlorophyll; in fact, molecularly they differ by only one molecule (magnesium in plants and iron in humans). By combining the water of one coconut and one ounce of wheatgrass juice with two ounces of beet juice (a great source of iron), a healing and rejuvenating drink can be made. This drink synthesizes almost 77 percent of human blood.

CITRUS

Citrus juice is extremely helpful in digesting old material, especially plaque and calcifications. Citrus is the sun bearer and offers a wide variety of vitamins (especially rich in vitamin C). Citric acid helps in the processing of fats and oils and can assist the liver in cleansing and help break down gallstones.

GRAPE

Grape juice is an excellent rejuvenator. Grapes can be juiced or ground in a Vita-Mix to produce a delicious juice with a delightful texture. Grapes are best juiced with their seeds (Concord grapes are some of my favorites). The grape seed is very high in picnogynols, a powerful antioxidant.

APPLE, CUCUMBER, AND KALE

Apples are abundantly rich in pectin and are very alkaline. Cucumbers are a vine fruit with many seeds containing large amounts of silica and magnesium, as well as high concentrations of organic sodium. Kale is a dark, rich, leafy green providing tons of iron and chlorophyll. This combo is great for people working on cleansing on a cellular level who want to avoid concentrated sugars. You can drink this juice two or three times a day with mild results to the digestive system and still provide yourself with an abundance of energy and nutrition. Combine one part kale juice with two parts apple juice and two parts cucumber juice. Stir and enjoy.

ALOE, LIME, AND CELERY

Aloe vera is a powerful healer and a member of the succulent family (a type of cactus). Aloe is extremely high in mucopolysaccharides and saponins. Aloe has very bitter taste, though the taste varies depending on the strain. Aloe vera juice is a wonderful detoxifier and flushes toxins from the bloodstream. Aloe also helps heal the lining of the stomach, which can get damaged by extreme acidity. The cells are made more permeable and can release intercellular toxins more easily after regular use of aloe vera juice. Lime is an excellent way to increase alkalinity, and the citric acid helps break down old fats, assisting the liver and gallbladder in their functioning. Celery, like cucumber, is a fantastic source of organic sodium and contains a good amount of chlorophyll. This combo, if made properly, is delicious and a strong way to rejuvenate the body from the cells to the organs. Combine three parts celery juice with one part aloe juice and one part lime juice. Stir and enjoy.

APPLE, CELERY, AND GINGER

Apples and celery are covered in the two previous juice combinations. Ginger is a fantastic bronchial aid and a vasodilator. That means that it helps open up the bronchi in the lungs, and the veins and capillaries are also widened. Ginger also increases internal heat and warms the body as well as helps to eliminate parasites and blood toxins. Combine four parts apple juice with four parts celery juice and one part ginger juice. Stir and enjoy.

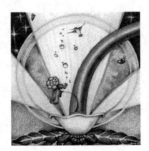

Soup

Fasting on soup is practiced by blending everything you consume. Soup fasting is excellent because you can do it for extended amounts of time. Soup in many ways is easier for the body to digest, since it is already fully masticated (chewed). When you are doing a soup fast, it is best to have a strong blender. It is a good idea to mix soup with salivary amylase in the mouth before swallowing and follow the adage "chew your drinks and drink your food." Salivary amylase is an enzyme found in human saliva that breaks down starch to sugar. It is very easy to come off a soup fast because you always keep your body working by giving it food. If you fast on soup for an extended amount of time—six months or many years—take at least twenty-eight days to move back into eating.

Soup Fast

	Breakfast	*Lunch*	*Dinner*
Day 1 in	Fruit	Blender soup	Soup
Day 2 in	Juice	Blender soup	Soup
Day 3	Choose a variety of soups and continue for as long as you choose.		
Day 1 out	Juice	Soup	Soup with avocado chunks
Day 2 out	Papaya	Soup	Soup with avocado chunks
Day 3 out	Papaya	Soup	Paté
Day 4 out	Fruit	Paté	Paté and avocado
Day 5 out	Fruit	Paté	Salad
Day 6 out	Fruit	Paté	Salad and sprouts

SENSATIONAL SOUPS

To prepare the following soup recipes, place all ingredients in a blender or Vita-Mix and pulse blend until the pieces are chopped up. Then blend until smooth and serve.

Tom Yum Ghai

2 cups fresh young coconut meat
2 cups coconut water
1 small hot pepper
1 inch of ginger root
1 cup mixed herbs (oregano, cilantro, basil, parsley)
3 teaspoons shoyu or salt

Dr. Ann's Energy Soup

1 ripe avocado
1 ripe papaya
1 handful of sprouts
2 tablespoons dulse flakes
1 tablespoon spirulina

Add water to blend.

Curried Cauliflower

2 cups diced cauliflower
1 large avocado or the meat of one coconut
1 small handful of cilantro
1 heaping teaspoon tahini
1 teaspoon honey
3 teaspoons Braggs Liquid Aminos or salt to taste
1 heaping tablespoon curry powder

Add water to blend.

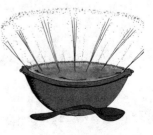

Carrot Ginger Soup

2 cups carrot juice
1 large ripe avocado
2 teaspoons Braggs or 1 teaspoon shoyu
1 small handful of parsley or cilantro
1 inch of ginger root

Pesto Soup

1 cup grated carrot and beet, mixed
1 cup tomato, diced
1 handful of dry walnuts
1 to 2 teaspoons miso
1 teaspoon nutritional yeast
2 sun-dried tomatoes, soaked
Pinch of onion
1 small clove of garlic
5 large basil leaves

Add water to blend.

Sprouts

Sprouts are one of the most powerful healers on the planet. Sprouts such as wheatgrass contain high amounts of chlorophyll and help carry oxygen throughout our body. Sprouts provide an abundant amount of life force and nutrition. It is excellent to eat sprouts that you have grown yourself. You can do a sprout fast by drinking green juice or sprout juice for two or three days, and then eat sprouts you have grown yourself to break the fast.

Sprouts are highly rejuvenating and bring vital nutrients to the cells. They also remove harmful toxins and free radicals from the body in safe and easy ways. Every seed, nut, bean, and grain is sproutable, and each sprout provides its own range of vitamins and minerals. It is a good plan to eat a variety of sprouts while fasting. Some of my favorite sprouts are sunflower, sesame, almond, buckwheat, garbanzo, and mung. Sprouts are the beginning of life for a plant and are bioactivated seeds. The seed is the plant's potential energy, and the sprout is that life force unleashed.

Sprout Fast

	Breakfast	Lunch	Dinner
Day 1 in	Fruit	Soup	Bowl of sprouts
Day 2 in	Juice	Soup	Bowl of sprouts
Day 3	Eat a variety of sprouts for as long as two weeks at a time. Create sprout drinks, soups, and salads.		
Day 1 out	Sprout juice	Sprout soup	Bowl of sprouts
Day 2 out	Sprout juice	Soup	Bowl of sprouts
Day 3 out	Juice	Soup w/ avocado chunks	Bowl of sprouts
Day 4 out	Juice	Kim chi	Sprout paté and avocado
Day 5 out	Juice	Paté	Salad and sprouts
Day 6 out	Smoothie	Paté	Salad and sprouts

Fruit

Fruit fasting is a fun fast where only fruit is eaten. Some fruit fasts are done as mono meals, eating only one fruit at a time. Other fruit fasts use many fruits in different combinations. Fruit fasting is suggested in warm climates where fresh fruit is available. Fruit fasts can be done for extended periods to allow the body and cells to cleanse themselves by bathing in clean organic water provided by the fruit. Organic water has an easier time entering and exiting the cell, thereby bringing nourishment into the cell and removing toxins efficiently. When fasting on a variety of fruit, it is good to maintain a balance of sweet fruits such as mangos, cherimoyas, and other tropical fruits with cucumbers, tomatoes, and melons. It is also excellent to eat fatty fruits such as olives or avocados to maintain protein and fat content while fasting. Multifruit fasts can be continued for lengthy periods such as one month to one year even if only one type of fruit is eaten at a time. Mono fruit fasts (one kind of fruit for the whole fast) are best done for three days to one month maximum. For further fruit suggestions, see my book *The Raw Truth,* (Ten Speed Press, 2003).

Fruit Fast

	Breakfast	*Lunch*	*Dinner*
Day 1 in	Fruit	Salad with avocado	Anything raw
Day 2 in	Smoothie	Fruit	Fruit salad with nuts
Day 3	Eat a variety of fruits or just one and continue for as long as you choose.		
Day 1 out	Fruit	Fruit	Fruit with nut kreme
Day 2 out	Fruit	Fruit	Fruit with nut kreme
Day 3 out	Fruit	Fruit with nut kreme	Veggie soup
Day 4 out	Fruit	Fruit with nut kreme	Veggie soup
Day 5 out	Fruit with nuts	Paté with avocado	Salad
Day 6 out	Fruit	Paté	Salad and sprouts

Nutrition (Living Food)

Fasting on nutrition is accomplished by consuming only food designed to provide the maximum amount of nutrition. Many foods these days are referred to as superfoods. These foods provide an abundance of vitamins, minerals, protein, fats, and carbs and usually have a tremendous amount of life force and energy. Sometimes the needs of your body can be met in a more efficient way. Nutritional deficiencies occur slowly as your body uses stores of nutrients. Providing concentrated nutrition lets your body store away what might be needed at a later date. Dr. Ann Wigmore is famous for saying that 85 percent of the nutritional value of food is destroyed by cooking it. That means that people eat eight to ten times as much food as they need in order to get the proper nourishment. By consuming food that provides maximum nutrition with minimum waste, you offer your body the opportunity to do less and be more effective. Some of the finest sources of nutrition are spirulina, bee pollen, kelp, hot peppers, sea vegetables, nutritional yeast, avocado, flaxseeds, hemp seeds, papaya, wheatgrass, sprouts, coconut water, green juices, and sprouted coconut.

In order to fast on nutrition, you consume only raw food. You eat as much from the above listed items as possible, and eat one to two meals a day of energy pudding. Nutritional fasting can be done for extended periods of time (one to six months).

Energy Pudding

In a food processor blend: 1 to 2 avocados, 1 hot pepper, 3 teaspoons spirulina or other algae, 3 teaspoons nutritional yeast, 1 pinch of Celtic sea salt, 1 teaspoon dulse or kelp, 1 teaspoon lemon juice, 1 teaspoon flax or hemp oil, and some fresh sprouts or green herbs. This can be eaten on flax crackers (made from ground flaxseeds and fresh herbs dehydrated).

The purpose of this fast is to bring concentrated nutrition into the body, and it is an excellent way to live and rebuild between cleanses or during a time of focused healing. (In and out times are not required as you continue to eat raw food the whole time.)

Alkaline Substances

Fasting on alkaline substances is a great way to bring the body into a more balanced state. Your body's pH helps regulate the way bacteria interact with your body. Often, because of overconsumption of starches, meat, dairy, and chemicals or through inhaling smoke or harmful vapors, your body can become highly acidic. One good way of telling your acidity level is to look into the iris of the eye (iridology), and if there is a large amount of white lines or flecks, this suggests an acid condition. Another method of testing is to use pH or litmus paper. An acidic body is much more likely to hold onto toxins than an alkaline body. Acidic bodies are the breeding ground for all types of parasites and also create an environment that allows cancer and immune deficiencies to prosper. By consuming alkaline water and alkaline-forming food, your body becomes healthier. Some examples of alkaline food are dry figs, dry apricots, raisins, Swiss chard, dandelion greens, soy sprouts, cucumbers, avocados, almonds, and kale.

Acidic Substances

Sometimes the body gets into an extreme alkaline state, which can cause energy deficiencies and can even cause internal organs to become soft and wet (too yin). This can lead to degenerative diseases such as Crohn's or diabetes. Certain food can bring the body back into balance and create an ideal state of homeostasis. Acidic-forming food includes Jerusalem artichokes, walnuts, wheat, olives, filberts, blueberries, peas, and watermelon.

To create an alkaline or acidic fast, consume mostly or only food that creates the ideal condition and avoid food that supports the unwanted condition.

Fasting From

Speech

Speech fasting is the practice of not speaking. This type of fast is very useful in learning to "think before you speak." Language can often get in the way of communication between people. When we look at our words internally instead of just talking, we can learn how to refine our speech and express ourselves to the fullest. Speech fasting lets us take a closer look at our own inner dialogue. Words have power. They are one of many ways that we can affect our world. Although it is advisable to do a speech fast alone, speech fasting can also be done in groups in order to create new ways of communicating. Speech fasting is also great when preparing for public speaking. It is wonderful to speech-fast the day before a big talk; it helps create greater clarity and allows us to be more concise.

SPEECH FAST

Choose a day when you feel you will be able to commit to silence. The night before you speech-fast, it is a good practice to let someone, such as a friend or fasting partner, know what you are planning. It is also a good idea to make any necessary calls the previous day. Before you go to bed on the eve of your speech fast, turn off your phone and make a clear sign, to be hung on the door of your home, stating that you are not to be disturbed.

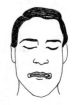

Media

A media fast is when you remove all TV, magazines, newspapers, radios, and advertisements from your life. Media fasting gives you a better insight into what is going on in your personal world. Many people focus on what is happening out in the world and miss out on what is right there in their own life. "The media" tries to fill our minds with fear-based illusions and spreads mostly rumors. In this day and age, there are so much hype and so many sales pitches that by exposing our minds to the media we are signing up for a program that may not lead to health. There is so much diversity and opportunity for growth in our own personal worlds that to spend any time thinking about the things we cannot change draws us away from changing the things we can. The microcosm always reflects the macrocosm. By making small changes in yourself and your world, the changes can resonate out and open up new possibilities in the big picture. The media only tells us what it wants us to hear and feeds us omens that lead to the outcome it expects. If you watch your own world and personal omens, you find your own dharma and see your life in a clearer way.

To fast from media, unplug all TVs and radios. Put away or throw away all newspapers and magazines and, when the mail comes, instantly throw away all junk or commercial mail (if you have really won $1,000,000, they will call you again). Go for a good amount of time, such as one month, or really go for it and give that program up all together.

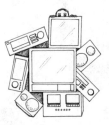

Sight

We take most of our information in through our eyes. The things you see influence you whether or not you are aware of it. Everything you see is recognized and recorded by your brain. Much of the stimulation in today's world has a program to it, and it may not be the best one for you. Visual stimulation causes people to do many things based on their relation to the imagery presented. By extracting yourself from the visual world of the outside, you get more in touch with your own visions and dreams. Your inner sight can teach you lots about yourself. Often during a sight fast, old imagery surfaces to help remind us of what may have been seen and may not have been noticed. There is a big difference between looking at something and really seeing it. Sight fasting can help repair damaged retinas and can also strengthen your hearing. When one sense is impeded, the others are strengthened. By keeping the eyes closed or wearing a blindfold, you can impede visual sensory stimulation and thereby rely on your other senses more.

Sight fasts are accomplished by keeping your eyes closed for anywhere from one hour to three days. Traditionally, sight fasts are done with a guide who helps lead you and can support you through this fast. There are cases where people have regained vision and gained the ability to see more after practicing sight fasting. Complete darkness helps produce human growth hormone and allows your glandular system to balance itself (mostly regulated by the pituitary). Get out your blindfolds and, remember, no peeking.

Sleep

Fasting from sleep is a great way to induce powerful dreams. Sleep fasting is like hitting the reset button on your dreamtime. When you sleep, you get into certain patterns of comfort. Your body gets used to getting the opportunity to detoxify your mental and emotional states in your dreams. Sometimes your dreamer gets caught in a repetitive pattern (reoccurring dreams) or offers reflections that you are unable to understand. Some dreams can even evoke fear and anxiety. It is important to remember that we spend one-third of our life in bed and some of that time dreaming. Your dreams can be great teachers and guides, as well as a testing ground to work things out or say or do things you don't or won't do in life. Choosing to stay awake when you normally would be sleeping offers new perspectives and can help you define new patterns of sleeping. When you take the day off from sleep, your mind compiles much of the information taken in. You will be able to see a clearer pattern running through your life because of the extra amount of sensory stimulation (two days' worth rather than one). When you finally sleep, your mind will give you a much clearer picture of what is going on and may help you uncover things from your past or present that have been challenging you. Dreams can offer excellent reflections on life. It is advisable to keep a dream journal and track your progress.

It is best to fast from sleep only once in a while (once a season, once a year) because the body does require sleep. Sometimes sleep fasting will make you sleep very deeply afterward and then bring your daily dosage of sleep down. Remember that meditation is very helpful in times of sleep fasting and can keep you from getting cranky because of lack of sleep. There are also herbs such as kava kava (vivid dreams) and valerian (for deep sleep) that can help us coming down from a sleep fast. Dream well.

People

There can be times when we need to be completely by ourselves. Time alone can give you an opportunity to reflect and come to a greater innerstanding. One of the greatest quests is the one of self-knowledge. Being with yourself gives you a greater experience of who you are. During these fasts from people, you get the opportunity to see what is truly you and what is programming from outside. Many patterns that we engage in daily may not be as deeply ingrained in us as we think. Some patterns are stimulated by the people around us. When you take a break from the people in your life who influence you, you gain the strength to break your patterns and transform your life.

The best way to do a people fast is to go camping or use a friend's house in the woods when they are away. It requires boundaries to do people fasting at home. Friends may unexpectedly drop by, or a phone ring may sound so interesting that you just have to pick up. Whatever the distraction, being at home may be challenging for people fasting. So get away from people, go somewhere quiet and peaceful, and be with yourself, your thoughts, and maybe your journal.

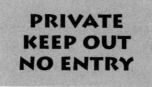

PRIVATE
KEEP OUT
NO ENTRY

Sex

Sometimes you need to rejuvenate the sex organs and nurture your healing in the area of sexuality. By taking a break from sex, you can gain new perspectives. There is a lot of pressure in modern society relating to sexuality. Taking a sexual time-out is a great opportunity to understand more about our own desires and feelings. Sometimes in a relationship you want to create greater closeness in other areas of intimacy besides sexuality. By removing sex from the equation for a bit of time, you can open up to new ways of relating to your partner. Many partnerships become too casual and often lose the beauty of the intimacy they started with. By fasting from sex, you renew your interest and gain new understandings that can be exciting and uplifting when you return to sexual interaction. Some sex fasts are performed by maintaining all intimacy with the exception of intercourse. Other sex fasts are practiced by creating no sexual desires or stimulation. In kung fu, there are many types of training that require all sexual energy to be transformed within the body in an internal alchemical process designed to create longevity and certain physical prowess. Sometimes going within through sex fasting can allow you to understand and remember things in your past relating to sexuality. Everything from abuse to past lovers may surface to offer us an opportunity to grow or just to remember and bask in the joy of intimacy.

Sex fasting is also a good way of conserving energy. When you interact so closely with someone else, you share little parts of yourself. By fasting from sex, you can be 100 percent yourself and really identify what that is. Transformation of sexual energy or internal alchemy is also one of the practices of the Taoists working toward immortality. In yoga, bramacharya is the focusing of the sexual energy upward for the purpose of enlightenment.

Water

Fasting from water is a strong statement. Water is necessary for life. In today's world, water may be more poisoning that healing. Some water travels through pipes that are made of copper, plastic, and sometimes lead or through pipes that are held together by lead solder. The toxins from these substances can leach into our bottled water and tap water. We also do not know what else is done to the water before it reaches us. Much of the bottled water you can buy is actually tap water from other places. Removing H_2O from the diet can only be done if you replace it with some other form of hydration such as coconut water, juice, or watery fruits. The body is an amazing mechanism. It can completely purify water for all your vital functions. Water fasting can be done for extended periods if the person fasting is in a moist environment and is getting other forms of hydration.

To fast from water, choose an appropriate amount of time (I went for three years without a single drop, drinking only coconut, orange, apple, watermelon, and panini juice instead). One week to one month is usually good. Then make certain that you will be able to obtain hydration from other plant-based sources.

This is not advised for people in desert or dry climates.

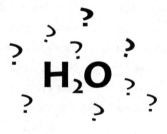

Sweet Foods

Many people consume far more sweets than their body requires. Sweet food is often a way of giving yourself a reward. These foods do invoke the pleasure principle and help us feel good by enjoying the sweetness of life. Sweets can bring you out of balance and cause a greater insulin response. Sweets are also a major contributor to the energy level of your body. The more sweet foods you eat, the more your body craves them. By putting sweet food aside for a week or two, you gain a better understanding of your body's craving and also get a chance to balance the sweet with the bitter. Foods such as kale, chard, spinach, parsley, burdock, and dandelion greens are great examples of bitter food. By eating these foods, your body adjusts, and when you return to eating sweets you may find that some foods are now too sweet. Sweet fasting is done by putting aside all sweeteners (honey, sugar, dates, maple syrup, fructose), all sweet foods (tropical fruits, sweet fruits), and high–glycemic value foods (potatoes, wheat, corn, rice, carrots).

Mucogenic Foods

Mucogenic foods are foods that cause an extreme mucous response in the body or create a large amount of mucus. Foods such as dairy products (milk, cheese, ice cream, and even skim milk), yeasted breads, and even soy can all cause an extreme mucous response. By eliminating these foods, you can begin to breathe again. Mucous will clog the intestines, the lungs, and even areas in between the muscles. Mucous is very sticky stuff and will limit your digestion, breathing, and ability to move. By removing these foods from the diet, we gain a new sensation of lightness and ease. Fasting from mucogenic foods is done by removing any food that creates mucus in your body. Some examples are listed earlier in this paragraph.

Chemicals

Fasting from chemicals takes great awareness. Modern society attempts to put chemicals in everything, so watch out. A chemical is any substance that has been created synthetically or manipulated to such an extent that it has no relation to the original substance. There are three types of minerals that exist: organic (plants and animals), inorganic (rocks and dirt), and synthetic (made by humans in a lab). Chemicals are in foods, in supplements, in shampoos, in soaps, in detergents, in beauty products, on clothing, on stamps and envelopes. Airborne chemicals are in spray cans and car fumes. Many chemicals are so new that we don't even know all the effects they may have. The best way to fast from chemicals is to go to nature and eat, drink, and breathe. Wear only natural fiber, organic clothing and use only natural house-cleaning and body-cleaning products. This type of fast can be done forever and however much your body appreciates it. The planet and future appreciate it more.

Seasonings

Seasonings are the things that make many foods into meals. Seasonings are flavor enhancers. Foods such as salt, Braggs, cayenne, garlic, many herbs, and anything we use in small amounts to affect the flavor of the things we consume are all seasonings. In modern times, many people have forgotten the true taste of foods. When we go for some time without seasonings, we begin to comprehend the true taste and flavor of foods. Seasonings are in almost all prepackaged foods. In order to fast from seasonings, it is best to make all your foods yourself or eat only whole foods. This type of fast can be done for any length of time.

Remember that variety is the spice of life, not salt.

Starchy Foods

Starchy foods are foods such as potatoes, corn, wheat, carrots, most grains, most roots, and all bread/flour products. These foods create a glycemic response and are often challenging for the liver and gallbladder. By avoiding starchy foods, your body has an easier time cleansing and healing the liver. Starchy foods also provide energy imbalances and can cause a variety of side effects from mood swings to lethargy. Fasting from starchy foods can be done for extended amounts of time (one to three months, even longer if advised).

Favorite Toxin

Fasting from your favorite toxin is often a nice change of pace. We all have vices or things that we do or consume that we know are less than excellent. If we can identify what they are and decide to put them aside for a while, we can gain new understanding about their place in our life. Many people smoke, drink, eat candy, or subject themselves to toxic environments or situations. If we take time away from these, we may break the hold they have on us. Our body craves certain substances for emotional, mental, or physical reasons. Putting our favorite toxin aside is a great way to gain personal power. Toxin fasting can be done by setting a realistic goal (one day, one week, one month, one year) and putting the toxin aside until the end of the fast, where you may want to reassess and continue or break your fast.

Work

Fasting from work is a great way to see what you have to offer the world rather than what is expected of you at your job. Work fasting means taking a vacation and really taking all doing, talking, and thinking time off. There are many projects (self-discovery most important of all) that we would all like to finish. When you take time out from the day-in, day-out rat race, you begin to accomplish your own personal destiny.

Practices for Cleansing

Lymph

The lymphatic system is one of the most efficient ways the body has to remove toxins. The blood deposits toxins into the lymph to be exited from the body through the urinary tract or by the sweat glands and the skin. The lymphatic system functions on gravity, always moving downward. The best way to assist the lymph in doing its job is by giving it a rest. This can be accomplished in a variety of ways. When we invert our body (go upside down), the lymph is given a chance to reduce pressure and balance itself. The best way to do this is getting on a slant board. The slant board is a bench that is at a 45° angle. Often a weight bench or even an old table with legs only on one side works well. Home slant boards are available from many sporting goods stores. Headstands, handstands, gravity boots, and inversion swings are all excellent methods of inversion. The second method of lymphatic cleansing is bouncing. When we jump up, the liquid in the lymph is suspended momentarily and this gives it a moment's rest. This is not as efficient as fifteen minutes of daily inversion, yet it is often beneficial. The third method is dry skin brushing. This method is covered under "Skin" in this section and under "Fasting Assistants." By keeping the lymph at its optimal level of function, we experience less detoxification reactions. This is due to the fact that by keeping the lymph working well toxins are removed at a more rapid rate. Many detox symptoms are the result of high concentrations of toxins in the bloodstream. When the lymph is clean, the blood can deposit toxins more rapidly into the lymph to be removed from the body.

Lungs

The lungs are the largest organ of detoxification. We exhale thousands of toxins per minute since our body uses respiration to remove much of the cellular waste. By cleansing the lungs, you increase your capacity for respiratory intake of nutrients and open space for cellular detoxification. The lungs are our connection to life. We are in a constant state of respiration, inhaling and exhaling the ebb and flow of the human body. We can go without food for weeks, without water for days, and without sleep for days, yet we can only go a few minutes without breathing. The lungs are filled with many bronchi. These are small passages where the blood is brought in tiny capillaries near the inner surface of the lungs. The bloodstream releases toxins through these bronchi into the lungs to be exhaled. The lungs are also coated with a thin mucous membrane where airborne toxins are trapped so as not to be let into the bloodstream. When toxicity is increased, or we begin to cleanse and detoxify, the amount of mucus in the body often increases as a protective measure.

The best way to detox the lungs is to breathe. Pranayama (yogic breath control) is one of the best ways to accomplish this (see the section on pranayama under "Fasting Assistants"). Any type of deep breathing or focused breath work will assist the lungs in doing their job more efficiently. There are many herbs such as lobelia, mullein, mugwort, sage, and ma huang that help the lungs expel toxins and act as expectorants and soothing agents. Singing, chanting, and toning can open up new areas of the lungs and help us let go of old toxic buildup. Increases in our respiration by aerobic activities also move toxins out of the lungs at a more rapid rate. Breath is life, so breathe well and live well.

Liver

The liver is responsible for cleansing the blood; it removes toxins and stores them safely until they can be removed. The liver is also in charge of glycogen storage, that is, sugar that the body converts and stores for later usage. The liver is often considered the top of the digestive system and therefore a great place to start the cleaning of the alimentary canal. Many people's liver is greatly enlarged and highly toxic from overconsumption of fried foods, cooked oils, and especially high–glycemic index starches like potatoes, wheat, corn, and rice. The liver is the hottest organ in the body and is often the hardest working. By cleaning the liver, we give our body the opportunity to have more energy and give us greater endurance.

The liver is cleansed by removing all high–glycemic index foods and heavy toxins such as alcohol, smoke, chemicals, and oils from daily intake. A juice fast on panini juice (lowest on the glycemic index) or a fast on watermelon juice including the rind can be helpful. Dandelion greens and parsley are also beneficial to the liver. Practicing a gallbladder flush alongside a liver cleanse can help reduce the liver's size and shorten the detoxification process. The liver is often put into peristalsis (contraction) by doing a coffee or wheatgrass enema. Castor packs on the liver can also be helpful. Drinking coconut water will give the liver the ability to clean the blood faster and easier. The liver is also very responsive to massage. By cleansing the liver, we allow it to do its job of helping us cleanse the rest of our body.

Gallbladder

The gallbladder is responsible for bile production. Most people produce hundreds of gallstones every year. These gallstones are made of rancid fats and oils and calcified minerals. Gallstones can be released naturally if you live a healthy lifestyle, but most gallstones get stuck and are stored in the gallbladder itself. Many people have gallbladders packed with stones. A gallbladder flush can remove blockages and expel stones. A gallbladder flush is accomplished by fasting for three to five days on lemonade, apple juice, and low–glycemic index blended soups. Do castor packs on the liver and gallbladder daily and massage the area. By breaking down the calcification using malic acid in apples, and by massage and castor packs, the exterior of the stones will begin to dissolve. On the day of the flush, fast on apple juice or water. The flush itself is done by drinking eight ounces of lemon juice and twelve ounces of oil. This is most easily achieved by drinking 2-oz. shots of oil chased by a 1.5-oz. shot of lemon juice. If you live a very clean lifestyle and your bowels move quickly, then you can use hemp or flaxseed oil or any oil that will not go rancid in under five hours. If this is your first flush or you are uncertain as to your digestion time, use olive oil. Olive oil has a very low rancidity rate and is quite heat stable (your body temperature is 98ºF). It is best to do the flush either at noon (you will pass your stones around 6 to 10 P.M.) or at 11 P.M. (you will pass your stones in the morning), although any time is acceptable. After drinking the oil, lie on your left side with a castor pack on your liver and gallbladder area. It is often nice to have a hot water bottle as well. Note that you may feel a bit queasy during this fast. Rest well all day and if in five to ten hours you have not passed stones, then do an enema either with coffee or with a wheatgrass implant. The stones will be greenish yellow to orange-brown and will float in the water.

Blood

In order to purify the blood, we must first look at what blood is. Human blood is primarily plasma, a clear substance that transports all our different blood cells and nutrients. Our bloodstream is 55 percent plasma. The next major constituent of blood is hemoglobin. Heme is our red blood cell, the carrier of oxygen. Heme is made of a variety of minerals, iron being one of the more prevalent ones. Hemoglobin makes up 22 percent of our blood. The rest of our blood is made from minerals, vitamins, sugar, oxygen, and white blood cells (the body's defense mechanism)

To cleanse the bloodstream, it is helpful to dilute our blood by consuming large amounts of a plasma analog. The best one is young coconut water, a substance nearly identical to blood plasma. In fact, in many countries intravenous medicine is given in a coconut water base. Coconut water is completely sterile and sealed in an organic container. If coconut water is not available, then very pure charged water can be transformed by the body. By consuming mass amounts of plasma analogs, the body can dump into the urine the toxins currently riding along in the bloodstream. To begin blood purification, choose a liquid fast such as the coco water fast or charged water fast. When the fast is in full swing (you are consuming only water), drink a quart of coco water first thing in the morning. Then drink one pint of coco water every hour, for about one to four hours, until your body is rapidly evacuating (urinating). At this point, begin to consume a pint of coco water with two teaspoons of wheatgrass or spirulina dissolved in it. Drink this mixture whenever hungry or thirsty. Do this cleanse once and for only one day during a fast.

Parasites

Everyone has parasites. The food we eat, water we drink or bathe in, the clothes we wear, the bed we sleep in, and especially places we go all contain hundreds of tiny parasitic organisms. A parasite is basically an organism that takes from our body and doesn't give anything back. It is important to cleanse parasites after exposure to food or water in foreign countries. There are many types of parasites affecting all areas of the body. Parasitic organisms avoid healthy bodies, so the cleaner your body and the greater abundance of healthy bacteria you have, the more likely that parasites will find your body an uncomfortable place to stay. If you have toxicity or illness in any way, it is likely that you have parasites. Constant hunger, continual loss of weight, lack of energy, and strange sensations in the organs all can be signs of potential parasitic invitation. Parasites can be removed in a number of ways. Fasting on onions and garlic (and any of the allium family) will expel a whole variety of parasites (especially liver, gallbladder, and intestinal parasites).The more blended or masticated the allium, the more effective they are, since the pungent qualities that surface when blended help create an unfriendly environment for parasites.

This allium fast is usually done for about a week to ten days. Food from the allium family can be eaten straight or in combination with other food. One of the best herbal combinations for expelling parasites is clove, quassia, papaya seeds, garlic powder, wormwood, and black walnut (consult an herbalist for combinations or see our order form). This combination is consumed for 100 days once or twice per day along with a healthy diet. Mini-allium cleanses can also be done during the 100-day period. Parasites can be fasted out of the body. When we lessen the amount of food we eat, parasites go hungry and decide to leave. Also, by increasing the alkalinity of our body, we create an unfriendly environment for the parasites. Consuming large amounts of cabbage and kim chi/sauerkraut can be helpful both during the fast (to create an antiparasite environment) and after (to rebalance flora).

Stomach

The stomach is the first organ that our food encounters when entering the body. The stomach is where we balance acidity and alkalinity and where enzymes become potent and begin the digestion of our food. The stomach is helped in its job considerably by chewing and by the mixing of food with salivary amylase. The stomach is one of the important organs to clean when making dietary changes. Eating more or only raw/living food or becoming vegetarian can be an extreme change for the body. Our body can be shocked by changing the type of food, or food of certain pH ranges, that the stomach is used to receiving, and this may cause discomfort. If we slowly transition into healthier eating, our body will have an easier time with the change. If you seek to change your diet more rapidly, the best thing you can do is practice cleansing and fasting to help the body in its transition.

The stomach is traditionally cleansed in yoga in one of two ways. The first is the drinking of saltwater, not seawater, and usually up to a gallon. This practice is usually done first thing in the morning and, after drinking the saltwater, it is vomited back up. This causes the body to expel many toxins trapped in the stomach and also helps reset the pH of the stomach. The other technique is the swallowing of a cloth. For this practice, seek out a yoga instructor familiar with the kriyas. Other ways of cleansing the stomach are the eating of raw honey, green papaya, and pineapple. All these foods are extremely high in enzymes and will make the body's job of breaking down food easier. This food will also help digest old material in the stomach and balance the pH. One of the best fasts for stomach cleansing is the lemonade or master cleanser fast. And always remember to chew well.

Kidneys and Bladder

The kidneys and bladder rule over the element of water within the body. The kidneys are responsible for filtering the blood. By offering our body extremely high quality water, we help the kidneys do their job more efficiently. Organic water from fruits and vegetables and especially coconut water (nearly identical to human blood plasma) are ideal substances to ease the kidneys' workload. The kidneys are affected by salt balance in the body. When the body contains organic sodium or pure salts, it gains the ability to store water in our cells and can help the kidneys. The kidneys also function as the battery for the body's energy. By cleansing our kidneys, we create the ability to store more energy. The bladder is where water that is to be removed from the body is stored.

The kidneys and bladder are cleansed by drinking large amounts of coconut water and vegetable juices high in organic sodium such as celery, cucumber, and seaweed. Cranberries are extremely helpful in the dissolving of kidney stones. Watermelon juice with the rind is also an excellent way of detoxifying the kidneys. When cleansing the kidneys (fasting on organic water), it is often ideal to remove all inorganic water and processed salts from the diet. Baths with salt and seaweed can help recharge kidney chi. While practicing kidney cleansing, it is helpful to add some force to the process of urination. When eliminating old material from the bladder, use the breath to push outward, helping expel and cleanse. Chi kung is also very beneficial to the kidneys in rebuilding and rejuvenating.

Spleen and Pancreas

Through overconsumption of processed sugars and high–glycemic index foods, the spleen can get overworked. By focusing on removing sugar from the diet and fasting on substances such as panini juice or sunchokes (Jerusalem artichokes), we can begin to balance the insulin production in the body. The times of day we eat and the order in which we eat can play a crucial role in the way the body responds to foods. By moving into a diet high in leafy greens and sprouts, the body can regain its ability to balance blood sugar on its own. One of the most useful things to consume during a spleen/pancreatic cleanse is licorice root. Licorice helps balance the triglyceride (salt/sugar balance) levels in the body and eases the job of the spleen. Jujube is another spleen balancing food.

Intestines

The intestinal tract is where we absorb most of our nutrition. The villi (finger-like projections in the intestines) are coated with healthy flora and help us assimilate the maximum amount from our food. Through overconsumption of bread, meat, and processed food (especially all that bubble gum swallowed in high school), the intestines get clogged with old nucrose material and fecal mucoid matter. Many people's intestinal tract is coated with a thick rubberlike substance that limits their ability to absorb nutrition. Colon cleansing easily detoxifies the large intestine. The use of chompers and other edible intestinal cleansers aids in the breaking apart of old material trapped on the walls of the colon. Processes like colonics or enemas are also beneficial in the removal of intestinal waste. Fasting on water or wheatgrass is ideal for cleansing the colon. It is crucial to reintroduce healthy flora both orally and rectally after cleansing the colon. Kim chee/sauerkraut juice is one of the best ways to build flora and increase digestive fire.

Skin

The skin is one of the ways the body will eliminate if the organs of elimination are overtaxed. Acne and other skin eruptions are often the result of toxic or overworked kidneys and liver. Both the kidneys and liver will use the skin to expel toxins if they cannot process them quickly enough. Our skin can also be a good guide to the health of our organs and how well they are functioning. The skin can be cleansed by first helping the organs of elimination do their job most efficiently. Dry skin brushing and exfoliation are ideal for removing old dead skin cells and toxins. Hot baths that open up the pores are also great for helping the skin eliminate. Applying substances such as honey or papaya skins can help areas of the skin needing cleansing. These foods can digest old proteinaceous waste and ease detoxification. Foods such as avocado or aloe vera can soothe the skin and help in the healing process. Morning sun and bathing in natural streams and rivers are some of the best ways to nourish and nurture the skin.

Eyes

The eyes are one of the most used parts of the body. A large amount of information and visual stimulation is taken in through the eyes. Visual toxins can affect the eyes. TV is one of the most toxic visual substances, and it is best to avoid TV if cleansing the eyes. Practicing gazing exercises on yantras (symbols), a candle flame, or fire can help the eyes. The eyes can also be helped by the use of rainwater or dewdrops. In the morning, put a few drops of dew or fresh rainwater in an eyedropper and drip them in the eye. Opening the eyes under the ocean can also help detoxify the eyes. A sight fast can bring new clarity to the vision. Wheatgrass juice can also help the eyes through rapid recovery and rebuilding.

Nasal Passages

The nasal passages are crucial for breathing and the filtering of air. The nasal passages allow us to breathe in a healthy way. By cleansing the nasal passages, we can make the greatest use of our voice, refine our breathing, and help regulate all our body's cycles. The nasal passages can be cleansed by using neti, a yogic kriya or cleansing practice. Neti is practiced by filling a small neti pot or kettle (bowls even work) with slightly salty water. The head is tilted sideways, and water is poured down one nostril and out the other. This is practiced on both sides. Then water can be poured down the nose and come out the mouth.

Ears

The ears are often in constant use. Silence is one of the greatest ways to cleanse the ears. If you live in a noisy place, the ears will certainly benefit from cleansing. A quiet place, such as a forest or mountaintop, will certainly help cleanse the ears. Sitting by rivers, listening to rainstorms, and hearing the wind whipping through trees are all excellent ways to rebalance the hearing and ease our ears. The ears can be healed by toning as well. By humming or oming specific tones, we can assist our ears in fine-tuning and create even greater hearing abilities. The ears are also the home for our vestibular sense or sense of balance and direction. By cleansing the ears, we also gain greater poise and ability to move. One of the best methods of cleansing the ears is to use earcones. Earcones are candles for the ears. These cone-shaped candles are used through a paper plate. The small end is put into the ear, and the wide end is lit. The cone creates suction and pulls toxins and wax and old residue out of the ear cavity, allowing for greater hearing and hygiene.

Custom-Tailored Fasts

Design and Structure

Fasts, like life, are always unique and different for each person. We are each our own experiment and have reached our current state of being through our own process. That is why each person's needs from a fast, or type of fast, may be different. The reasons why we fast are the first things to consider. Is this a spiritual fast? If so, are we looking for a fast to challenge us and develop our sense of will and self, or is it for spiritual purification? Is this a fast to bring us power or to remove old things from our life? Is this a fast because we are working with a specific health challenge? Is this a maintenance fast or a deep cleansing? Each of these questions helps us define the ideal path for us to follow to our supreme health and well-being.

Always follow the carpenter's adage, "measure twice and cut once." Planning makes a lot of difference. It is vitally important to plan our fasts well and to be prepared. Make certain you will have the time to complete your fast in the way you want. Be certain that you have all the supplies you will need (seeds to sprout, clean water, journal, food supplies). Have a good idea of how you will break your fast (the most important part). With fasting, it is often good to test the waters before going in too deep. Daylong fasts or fasts that offer minor (as opposed to radical) change are a good way to get comfortable with fasting. When you are ready, create a fast that is most ecological (ideally, this means eating foods in season, local, and friendly to the environment) and economical (you can afford it—time and money). Fasting is a practice and a process that can yield different results for different people. Self-knowledge is the key. If we truly understand what we need the most, we can give it to ourselves in the best way possible.

Suggested Order of Cleansing

Cleanse the mind before the body.

By cleansing these organs/systems first, the body has the ability to process toxins out more rapidly.

LUNGS	GALLBLADDER
LYMPH	KIDNEY
LIVER	SKIN

Next, focus on areas that need cleansing. If you know you have a challenge or a hereditary tendency toward a particular organ or area, it is best to focus there.

STOMACH	NASAL PASSAGES
EARS AND EYES	SPLEEN AND PANCREAS

Next, focus on areas into which many toxins are washed or eliminated.

BLOOD	INTESTINES

Finally, return to cleansing the organs that help process toxins.

LUNGS	GALLBLADDER
LYMPH	KIDNEY
LIVER	SKIN

Fasting Assistants

Sleep

Light exercise

Chi kung

Pranayama

Yoga

Walks in the woods

Massage

Colon care

Deep breathing

Sun

Castor packs

Sweats

Slant boarding

Baths

Skin brushing

Meditation

Writing

Soothing music

Reading

Love

Rest and relaxation

Remembering

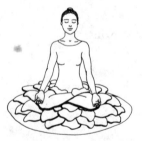

Sleep

Our body heals far faster in a relaxed state. When we sleep, the cells of our body heal and grow at a rapid rate. Sometimes dreams also help us detoxify experiences by assisting our mind in the recall of past emotions. When beginning a fast, we often sleep longer. As the fast progresses, we begin to become clearer and require less sleep. On some fasts, only four hours of sleep per night are necessary. When we sleep, we are lying down, and it is easier for our heart to pump blood throughout our systems. We can experience many great changes overnight. Often when we are unwilling to process something in our waking life, we take the opportunity to work it out in dreamtime.

When detoxing and transitioning into a new diet or lifestyle, many people will have memories or sensations of eating food or doing the exact thing that they are looking to extract from their life. This is an excellent sign, and it is often in these times that we are challenged and can learn about ourselves. Sleeping is a way of nurturing the body. As babies and children, we are allowed the time and space to sleep as needed so we can grow as much as possible. Cell replication doubles when we sleep. Staying in bed when fasting is a great way of offering our body a space that is warm, safe, and comfortable for cleansing and detoxifying.

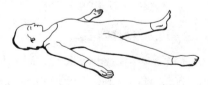

Light Exercise

When fasting, our body is spending most of its energy healing and cleansing. Exercise is used to build and add to our body. Any type of extreme exercise during fasting may cause our body to weaken and use up stores of energy unnecessarily. There is a time for all things, and fasting isn't usually a time for bulking up or lifting that extra twenty pounds. Heavy workouts (multiple hours of continuous activity, weight lifting, sprinting, marathons, lap swimming, or even powerful forms of yoga and kung fu) are usually put aside during fasts and cleanses. Each person is unique and will do what her or his body says is appropriate. Some people fast specifically to run a little faster or be a little more focused for a sporting event. These fasts are usually no longer than two days because of the extreme nutritional demands of the body after completing such a task. The following are a few examples of light exercise that will not overly stress the body and will still maintain good muscle tone and strength. Remember to work out less than one-third of your normal capacity in order to maintain your energy.

Jumping

Jumping, such as trampolining (a.k.a. rebounding), jump roping, and jumping jacks are excellent ways to stay fit and assist the lymph system in the cleansing process. Five to fifteen minutes per day are recommended.

Speed Walking

A nice fast-paced walk can help clear the head and maintain body tone. Flat, easy surfaces and comfortable distances (close to home) are ideal. It is best to stop before perspiring. Fifteen to thirty minutes per day are recommended.

Juggling

Learning to use your mind in new ways while exercising the body is great. Juggling teaches us to think with both sides of our brain and is a nice mellow form of exercise. Five to ten minutes per day are recommended.

Chi Kung

Chinese internal kung fu or energy work exercises are known as chi kung. These are exercises that train the body through focus, breath, and movement. Energy is circulated through the meridians, especially the governing and conception vessels. A wide variety of styles of chi kung are intended to achieve diverse purposes. As a continued disciplined practice, chi kung can create greater health and longevity as well as increase learning capacity, build strength and resilience, and even focus energy to help heal others.

Chi kung is often practiced in horse stance. The toes are pointed forward, feet are shoulder width apart, knees are slightly bent, and the spine is held erect. This is what is known as a light horse stance. Chi kung can also be practiced seated, lying down, and even while doing activities. The hands are usually in what is known as hugging a tree position, held out in front of the body, fingers facing fingers, thumbs facing thumbs, palms toward the body, elbows toward the earth, with a nice round space between your body and your arms. As you stand there, breathe in and concentrate on moving energy up your spine (governing vessel). As you exhale, focus on the energy moving down the front of your body (conception vessel). It is important to remember to have your tongue pressed onto the roof of your mouth and your bhandas (the Sanskrit word for *locks*) held locked. Part of the purpose of chi kung is to act as meditation to allow you to empty yourself, to know yourself, and to purify yourself. It is ideal to practice chi kung in a nice environment such as a forest, a river's edge, a beach, your room, a temple, or any place that is special to you. By circulating your energy, you can achieve a greater sense of balance and inner peace. Chi kung also allows you to assimilate energy and sustain fasts for far longer. By practicing chi kung while fasting, you fill the body with something other than food.

Pranayama

These are yogic breathing exercises designed around a number of purposes.
We detoxify very rapidly through the lungs. By practicing pranayama, the
nasal passages and bronchi of the lungs open up and allow for more rapid
detoxification. Pranayama is also a type of energy work like chi kung. By
focusing prana (energy) through the nadis (channels), we can awaken our
kundalini. Pranayama helps cleanse the sinus cavities. A wide number of
benefits are gained by practicing pranayama. Posture can play a key role in
our breathing. When practicing pranayama, it is best to hold the spine erect.
Often lotus or a kneeling pose is used for pranayama practice.

The following are two basic pranayama exercises.

Yogi Complete Breath

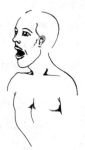

1. Sit comfortably.

2. Exhale all the air in your lungs.

3. Inhale smoothly and evenly, filling first the
    bottom, then the middle, and then finally the
    upper section of your chest cavity.

4. Now, exhale at the same rate that you inhaled,
    first from the upper section of the chest bot-
    tom, then the middle, and finally the bottom.

This may be practiced three or more times in a sitting.

Alternate Nostril Breath

1. Sit with good posture.

2. Hold the left hand in your lap; the right hand makes a mudra (hand position) by folding the ring and middle fingers in and holding the thumb near the right nostril and the ring and pinky fingers by the left nostril.

3. Exhale all the air in your lungs.

4. Close the right nostril and inhale through the left.

5. Close the left nostril and exhale through the right.

6. With the left nostril closed, inhale through the right.

7. Close the right nostril and exhale through the left.

8. Continue switching nostrils eight or more times.

Yoga

Yoga means union and is a path or group of paths that helps practitioners or yogi/yogini to achieve greater union with self and spirit. Yoga's limbs or paths are eight in number. They are Yama, Niyama, Asana, Pranayama, Pratayahara, Dharana, Dhyana, and Samadhi.

Yama and Niyama describe ways of living. Asana means pose or posture and is what is traditionally practiced as yoga in the West. Pranayama is the breath practices described earlier, and Pratayahara, Dharana, and Dhyana are types of meditation. Samadhi is a superconscious bliss state that is achieved by devoted yoga practice.

Yoga asanas can be highly beneficial during a fast. The movement and flexibility exercises help loosen up old toxins stored throughout the body. Many of the yoga practices can also help massage the internal organs and assist us in our cleansing process. There are many styles of yoga asana practice. Some are active, and others are more passive. On powerful cleanses, lighter forms of yoga are suggested; otherwise, practice whatever kind of yoga you feel most drawn to. The poses that most encourage cleansing are forward bend, shoulder stand, headstand, child pose, downward dog, and spinal twists. One of the most important things in yoga is the salutation to the sun. This practice is often used to warm up. It is the first thing practiced upon rising for many yogis around the world. If nothing else, the sun salutation itself makes an excellent daily yoga practice. It is suggested to practice it three to each side (six) or more times.

Surya Namaskara (Salutation to the Sun)

Stand with your hands in prayer in front of your chest.

1. Inhale and reach and look up.

2. Exhale and lean over, placing the palms flat on the ground (or reaching as far as feels comfortable).

3. Inhale, stepping back with the left foot, leaving the right foot planted, chest on leg and looking up.

4. Exhale, pressing the right leg back and bringing the knees and chin down to the floor.

5. Inhale while pressing up, keeping the knees off the floor, with the chest forward and eyes looking up.

6. Exhale and bring your head toward the floor, pelvis up into the air, and press the heels into the ground.

7. Inhale there.

8. Exhale there.

9. Inhale, stepping forward with the left foot as in #3.

10. Exhale, stepping forward with the right foot and leaning over as in #2.

11. Inhale while reaching and looking up.

12. Exhale and bring your palms into prayer in front of your chest.

Prayer to the Sun

Om Suryam Sundaralokanathamamritam Vedantasaram Sivam,
Jnanam Brahmamayam Suresamamalam Lokaikachittam Svayam;
Indradityanaradhipam Suragurum Trailokyachudamanim,
Brahmavishnusivasvarupahridayam Vande Sada Bhaskaram.

— SRI NAMASKARA

*I always adore Surya, the sun, the beautiful lord of the world, the immortal, the
quintessence of the Vedanta, the auspicious, the absolute knowledge, of the form of
Brahman, the lord of gods, ever-pure, the one true consciousness of the world itself, the
lord of Indra, the gods and men, the preceptor of the gods, the crest-jewel of the three
worlds, the very heart of the form of Brahma, Vishnu, and Shiva, the giver of light.*

Salutation to the Sun

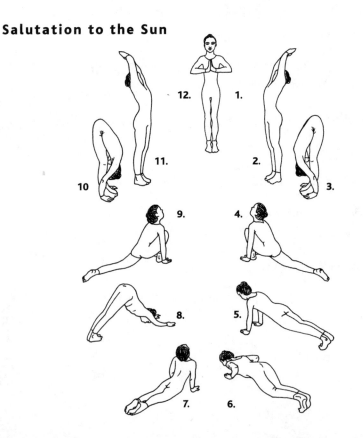

Walks in the Woods

Nature is one of the greatest healers. The answer to every question can be found in nature. By enjoying nature as much as possible, we are filled with the blessings of the earth. In a city, people with plants in their home lead far healthier lives than those without. Living in a natural environment is one of the best things that can be done for health and well-being. Walking in the woods gives us many opportunities to be exposed to information in its raw form. Everything we currently know was at one time based on nature and our experiences there. Walking in the woods can offer us solutions and ideas without any opinions. In societal interactions we find our reflections, and in nature we find ourselves. Walking is a nice way to relax, and nature offers so much. The leaves, flowers, seeds, animals, dirt, streams, and weather all inspire us and help us get back to our roots. The woods can also be a place of medicine, offering us what we need. A feather, a rock, a piece of fruit, or another person can all be part of the medicine we find in the woods. Getting away from our home and day-to-day environment can also help us in our detoxification.

Massage

Therapeutic touch is highly beneficial. By massaging the muscles and organs, we bring greater blood flow to the area and allow for more rapid detoxification. Massage also brings our awareness to certain areas of our body. Where our attention goes, energy flows, and we help our body heal. Massage can break apart toxic debris stored in the muscle tissue of the body. Massage is also very healing for the emotional body. By being touched in a healing way, we can get to places in our body/psyche and realize our issues and begin to release them. Massages can range from relaxing to invigorating. Find the style of massage that suits you the best. Or try a variety for different effects.

Colon Care

The colon or intestinal tract is where most of our nutrition is assimilated into our body. The intestines are coated with villi (little fingerlike projections that extend inward and are covered with healthy bacteria that assist in assimilation of food and protect us from foreign bacteria). The colon is part of the alimentary canal, a single tube starting at our mouth and ending at our anus. Food is transferred down this tube by peristalsis (tiny ripples in the muscles) and assisted by a coating of healthy mucus. The colon can get impacted with nucrose material and old unwanted matter. Often dead food, such as animal products, very starchy breads and crackers, and strange substances like chewing gum or marshmallow fluff, can get stuck in the intestines and will stay there for many years unless removed through cleansing. There are a great number of ways of cleaning the colon. Some methods such as colonics, cholemas, and enemas attempt to wash out the colon using hydrotherapy (water). Other techniques involve substances that will bulk-up and scrub-brush the colon. There is even food that is naturally laxative, causing intestinal release. The faster's motto is, "better out than in," and colon cleansing supports that. Many substances we haven't seen in years may surface as we clean the inside of our colon.

It is vitally important to remember to reseed our intestines with healthy bacteria after cleaning them. The healthy intestinal flora that live inside can be cleansed away during colonic therapy and can cause future complications. After any type of colon cleanse, it is a good idea to consume large amounts of acidophilus- and bifudus-rich foods such as cabbage, kim chi, sauerkraut, seed cheeze, rejuvelak, miso, amazake, yogurt, and so forth. It is also advisable to implant healthy bacteria if colonics, cholemas, or enemas were a part of your cleanse (see "Implants" later in this section). Most of our bacteria originally came from breast milk. Radiation, antibiotics, and poor diet can destroy our healthy bacteria, leaving us open for unfriendly bacteria. Be protected and remember that the best defense is a good offense.

Colonics

Colonic therapy is a practice used to cleanse the large intestine from end to end and ideally open up the iliosequal valve, which connects the large and small intestines. Colonic therapy is also known as a "high colonic" because it does cleanse the entire colon. A colonic is pressurized water that is flooded into the bowels and then sucked back out. Colonics and enemas both go against the body's natural process and create reverse peristalsis and over extended periods will weaken the body until it requires assistance in order to eliminate. It is advised to do colonic therapy only once in a while (once or twice a year, an intensive program of five to ten colonics over a twenty to thirty day period every three years, or at least once in your life). Colonics can be very helpful to those in extreme situations of health crisis. Colonics can rapidly remove toxic matter from the body and help us on a path to recovery. Colonics can help expel a greater volume of toxins at a more rapid rate. This can be very beneficial while going through a detox program where many intercellular toxins are surfaced and are best removed from the body as fast as possible. Colonic therapy is best done with a practitioner.

Enemas

Enemas are another method of cleansing the intestinal tract. Enemas only wash out the lower part of the large intestine. Enemas are easier on the body than colonics and can be done more frequently. With continued use, enemas can have the same or similar side effects as colonics. Enemas are done with anything from a gourd and vine to a plastic enema bag bought at your pharmacy. Enemas are gravity fed and cannot create very much pressure so will rinse only the surface toxins, unlike the colonic, which can go deep.

Cholemas

This is a type of colonic that was developed for home use. It cleanses deeper than an enema, yet not as well as a true colonic. Cholema boards hook onto the toilet (some on bathtubs) and allow for an easier experience. Cholema boards are simple to use and are very clean and hygienic. Many have ways to add implants.

Implants

When cleansing the colon, many healthy things are washed away with the old material. By implanting good flora such as acidophilus back into the intestine, we help our body recover faster and will have an easier time going back to eating after a fast. Healthy flora is seeded in our intestines at birth. Antibiotics and unhealthy bacteria cause our healthy flora to die. By implanting flora, we also strengthen our immunity. Wheatgrass is also something people will implant for a variety of reasons. One is that wheatgrass is very nutritious, and while fasting it can be easier on the body to absorb nutrition directly through the colon. Wheatgrass provides a wealth of cleansing benefits as well. It can help dissolve old fecal mucoid matter and detoxify the colon. Wheatgrass implants will also cause a peristaltic response in the liver. Herbs can also be implanted by making a tea.

Intestinal Massage

The intestines can have large amounts of waste matter clogging them and mucoid material stuck to the walls. By massaging the intestinal area, we can help break apart old material and assist the body in eliminating it.

Chompers

These are types of intestinal cleansers that are eaten or drunk. Chompers are usually a combination of herbs including psyllium husks and other bulking agents used to help push old material out of the intestines. Cassia pods and other laxatives can promote elimination by stimulating the bowels to move. If using these substances, it is advisable to be near a restroom. Make certain your bowels move daily when using chompers.

Deep Breathing

Breath is the key to life. We can go months without sunlight, weeks without food, days without water, yet only minutes without breathing. We detoxify many substances through our lungs and our breath. By breathing deeply, we can increase the rate of detoxification. Our lung capacity expands the more we practice deep breathing. The breath can also be a great form of nutrition. Some people are known as breatharians because they get much of their nutrition from deep breathing. Many micronutrients are airborne. Breathing deep is accepting and receiving the air that is our birthright.

Sun

Sunlight is nature's first medicine. The sun provides all of the energy for almost every life form on the planet. When dry fasting, it is excellent to get lots of sun (avoiding 11 A.M. to 2 P.M.) as long as you are in a moist environment (like the jungle). If you are fasting in a desert, always have supervision and avoid the sun. The sun is a brilliant ball of hydrogen, the simplest element. Exposure to the sun (especially full-bodied exposure) helps our body absorb nutrients like vitamin D, calcium, as well as a wide range of other nutrients.

Castor Packs

Castor packs are an excellent way to loosen up toxins and bring greater elasticity to the organs. Soaking a flannel or cotton cloth in castor oil creates a castor pack. Oil is rubbed on the area being cleansed and healed, and then the pack is applied on top of it. Many people wrap the area with plastic wrap to hold the castor pack in place and to keep from getting oil everywhere. Then a hot water bottle (often wrapped in a towel or cloth) is put on top of the pack. Castor packs can be done daily for one to twelve hours. When using castor packs, it is best to change them every four to six hours. This can be done once or twice a day.

Sweats

Our body can eliminate many toxins through the skin. As stated in the section on skin, the body will use the skin as an area of elimination. By helping the skin sweat, toxins can be expelled at a more rapid rate. Sweats can also help remove toxins trapped in the skin. One of the best ways to sweat is to take a hot bath or shower and then wrap up in a few sheets and get under some blankets. This will cause the body to sweat without getting too hot. Traditional methods such as exercise work well as long as the fast is not too extreme. Sweat lodges and saunas are also good ways to promote elimination.

Slant Boarding

A slant board is a plank at a 45° angle and is designed to help the lymphatic system eliminate toxins easier by creating slight inversion. A slant board is used by placing the feet up and the head down. Usually slanting is done for fifteen minutes. To avoid vertigo, come off a slant board slowly. Slant boards can be purchased or are easy to make with bricks and boards or even phone books and your bed. Slanting is an easy way to accelerate detoxification.

Baths

Baths are an excellent way of relaxing and healing. Our body is made mostly of water, and, when we fully submerge ourselves, we take the weight and pressure off many sore joints and tense muscles.

Herbal Baths

Herbal baths can help infuse our body with nutrients absorbed through the skin. Herbal baths can also encourage greater amounts of detoxification. When using herbs in a bath, it is often nice to put the herbs in a small bag or cloth to help contain them. Otherwise, you are welcome to add the herbs into the bath water directly. Yet another method is to make a tea of the herbs and add that to the bath water. Some excellent combinations are:

RELAXING: sage, rose petals, and lavender flowers.

MILDLY INVIGORATING: mint, eucalyptus, and vanilla.

VERY STIMULATING: ginger and hot peppers.

VERY MELLOWING: St. John's wort and valerian.

VERY HEALING: clay, spirulina, and seaweed.

EXTREMELY NUTRIFYING: wheatgrass and aloe vera.

Salt Baths

Salt baths give our body an opportunity to relax to an even greater extent. Saline water causes us to float and thereby lessens the amount of pressure on our organs and joints. Salt baths can soothe sore muscles and help diminish bruising. Sea salt is suggested, and often crystals can be added as well.

Skin Brushing

Dry skin brushing is an ideal way to rid the body of unwanted toxins. Skin brushing allows the lymphatic system to cleanse itself with ease and removes unwanted dead skin cells through exfoliation. Dry skin brushing is practiced by using a dry, natural-bristled brush on dry skin. Brush inward from the feet and hands, toward the heart. Five to ten strokes in each area (foot, shin, thigh, abdomen, fingers, forearm, arm, chest) on both sides of your body are sufficient. After skin brushing, it is good to bathe and rinse off any unwanted toxins.

Meditation

Meditation is a great way to stay centered and learn about ourselves. Meditation can also be helpful in cultivating internal energies. There is a wide variety of meditation. Some kinds involve sitting and allowing thoughts to pass through our head, others use focusing practices, and still others are all about keeping an empty mind. Meditation can allow us to cleanse concepts and experiences that may be causing us stress and helping keep toxins in the body. By meditating, we can often gain new perspectives and release old negative, false, and limiting concepts. Meditation is a way to distance ourselves from the judgments and projections of our mind. Often we carry other people's ideas of who we should be or how we should act. Teachers, parents, friends, and lovers all play parts in how we shape our consciousness. By meditating, we are effectively getting in touch with where our concepts come from. Through self-acceptance and innerstanding, we can take up power that we may have left tied up in the past. With a renewal of our integral self, we gain rebirth and cleansing. Some might consider meditation fasting from the mundane and material world.

Writing

Fasting is a time to let things come out, to detoxify our mind as well as our body. When we stop putting so much information into our mind, many more things will come to the surface. Our self-expression is key to our understanding of our inner nature. While fasting, working with a journal can keep track of thoughts and expressions. Also, writing exercises are a fabulous way to learn more about yourself (see writing exercises that follow). Another form of written self-expression is stream-of-consciousness writing, where you allow yourself to just flow with whatever your mind brings to the surface. Subject writing is where you choose a topic and write on that, such as: write about your last birthday or write a letter to yourself in ten years. Writing is a great marker of the past. We can look back upon our writing and see a glimpse of ourselves and who we were. Writing and drawing relax the mind and bring us deeper into ourselves. Pick a pen and a journal that you will enjoy and personalize them in some way and express yourself.

Here are some examples of writing exercises:

- Write the ten things you want to learn most.
- Write ten things you like about yourself.
- Write ten things you enjoy eating.
- Write ten things that make you smile.
- Write ten things you would like to leave behind.
- Write ten things you would like to create for your future.
- Write ten things you say the most.
- Write the names of the ten most influential people in your life and how they have affected you.
- Write a letter to someone you haven't spoken to in five years or more.
- Write a letter to yourself about your fast.
- Write a letter to yourself and give it to a friend to mail to you in five years to see how much you have changed.

Soothing Music

Anything that can help us relax, release, and rejuvenate is helpful during a fast. Music can be useful in helping us keep our center and hold our space while cleansing toxins. Relaxing, soothing music can help us feel more at ease while going through our process. Music is also a form of food. It has been said that music is food for the soul. Music does uplift and inspire as well as encourage and empower people. By listening to music, we may allow our body to cleanse in a comfortable way. Any way we can input positive information into the body to help clear out the old is beneficial.

Reading

Books and information can be quite useful while fasting. Sometimes we need encouragement, and there are many people who have cleansed and healed before us. Their testimonials can inspire us to cleanse and purify ourselves. Stories can also help us occupy our time while cleansing (don't mistake being distracted from internal processes for entertaining or educating oneself). It is best to read books that will uplift you. Sometimes reading books from the past can help surface memories from long ago and assist in detoxifying the body. Reading is a gathering of information and knowledge and is food for the brain.

Love

Love is probably the most important thing you can get. Love from family, friends, pets, spirit, and especially yourself is powerful medicine. Love may really be all you need. By receiving love, we can go farther, do more, and achieve what many deem undoable. Love is the greatest food there is and the most important ingredient in any meal. If there is one thing in this book that is most beneficial to everyone on a fast or cleanse, it is *LOVE*.

Rest and Relaxation

Getting rest is one of the most powerful ways to let the body do its job of cleansing and healing. When we stop "doing," our body's natural ability to balance and rejuvenate kicks in. Rest is the key to a successful fast. When we stay active during a fast, our body allows only a small amount of cleansing to occur. Our body heals the most when sleeping or in a deep state of rest. When we empty ourselves of our day-to-day "busyness," we can truly find our self and be ourselves. Relaxing by a river, sitting in a hammock, or just lying in bed all day are all excellent ways to relax and recuperate. People spend enormous amounts of energy on their daily struggle. When we fast, we want all our energy focused on healing.

Remembering

Going back through old journals and photo albums can help us recollect the past and gather up lost pieces of ourselves. We may surface some emotion or idea that we have been carrying since long ago. By remembering and recognizing what we were and where we came from, we can gain greater respect for others and ourselves and can also let go of the past by acknowledging the past as our teacher. Remember that the past is today's memory, and tomorrow is today's dream.

Self-Empowerment Questionnaire

Please answer the questions in the following questionnaire as accurately as possible. Write any information that seems applicable on the back of the questionnaire. Answer only the questions you feel comfortable answering. Any information provided will be kept confidential, help us in diagnosing you better, and help you in understanding more about yourself. It is useful to answer these questions every six months to track yourself and to understand your progress. Questions help us define ourselves and our beliefs and get us to think about choices.

The following is a questionnaire designed to track and gauge the process of healing. It is always best to take account of the situation before beginning a quest. By using this questionnaire monthly or yearly, progress can be tracked, and we can look at the results of the things we are doing with ourselves. Many of these questions are designed to make you think. If you don't know an answer, then take time and track yourself and come back to the questionnaire when you know yourself better. Every answer is correct because it is each individual's personal truth. By asking good questions of others and ourselves, we can learn the most and be highly empowered.

Send this questionnaire in to Loving Foods (see mailing information on page 85) with a self-addressed, stamped envelope, and we will advise you as to what type of fasting program or other practices would be best for you. We also set up custom retreats and yoga/chi kung practices for people.

- *$20.00 for a mail or email response*

- *$50.00 for a reading over the phone*

- *$188.00 for a personal consultation (first session)*

- *$108.00 for a personal consultation*
  Personal sessions include pulse diagnosis and iridology reading.

Name_____ Date of birth_____

Point of origin_____

Address_____

City_____State_____Zip_____

Phone_____ Cell/Work #_____

Email_____

Diet

How many meals do you eat per day? _____

How much time is spent at each meal? _____

What time of day are your meals eaten?

Breakfast _____ Lunch _____ Dinner _____ Other _____

How would you classify your diet or style of eating?

_____

Are you a vegetarian? (Y/N) How long? ____ Percentage of raw food in diet ____

Do you eat? (check all that apply)

❏ Meat	❏ Fruit	❏ Chocolate
❏ Eggs	❏ Vegetables	❏ Alcohol
❏ Dairy	❏ Sprouts	❏ Coffee
❏ Sugar	❏ Exotic fruit	❏ Fried foods
❏ Antibiotics	❏ Living cultures	❏ Coconut water
❏ Water	❏ Salt	❏ Chemicals

To what capacity of stomach fullness do you eat?

❏ 10 percent   ❏ 50 percent   ❏ 100 percent

❏ 25 percent   ❏ 80 percent

List your ten most favorite foods.

1._____   6. _____

2._____   7. _____

3._____   8. _____

4._____   9. _____

5._____   10. _____

List your ten least favorite foods.

1._____   6. _____

2._____   7. _____

3._____   8. _____

4._____   9. _____

5._____   10. _____

List the five healthiest foods you eat.

1._____   4. _____

2._____   5. _____

3._____

List five raw foods that you enjoy.

1._____   4. _____

2._____   5. _____

3._____

Meals are most often eaten (alone/with company)?

Do you read the ingredients on packages? (Y/N)

Do you like to try new things? (Y/N)

Do you prepare your own food? (Y/N)

Do you grow your own food? (Y/N)

Do you fast? (Y/N) How often? _____ For how long?_____

What kinds of fasts?

_____

_____

_____

Why?_____

_____

Body Practices

Do you practice yoga? (Y/N) What kind(s)? _____

What kind of exercise do you get? _____

How much time do you spend exercising? _____ daily _____ weekly

How far do you walk in a day on average? _____ Do you run? (Y/N)

How much of the time are you sitting? _____ How much standing? _____

Are you disabled in any way? (Y/N) Describe _____

_____

Since when? _____

Do you get sore? _____ How soon after you work out? _____

Do you smoke? (Y/N) How much?_____ What kind?_____

Are you healthy? (Y/N) Define health. _____

_____

_____

Emotions

How often do you cry? _____ How often do you yell? _____

How often do you laugh? _____ How often do you smile? _____

How often do you tell someone you love them? _____

How often do you think about death? _____ What specifically do you

think about with regard to death? _____

How do you feel? _____

_____

Are you emotionally balanced? _____

_____

If you were a color, what would it be? _____

How well do you express yourself? _____

_____

What ways do you express yourself? _____

_____

Do you hear music in your head? _____ What kind? _____

_____

Do you have pets? (Y/N) What kind(s)? _____

Who is the most significant being in your life right now? _____

Sexuality

How often do you make love? _____ How often do you ejaculate? _____

Are you (monogamous/polygamous)? _____

Are you celibate? (Y/N)

Are you (heterosexual/homosexual)? _____

Are you (married/divorced/single)? _____

Do you masturbate? (Y/N) _____ How often?_____

Do you enjoy sex? (Y/N) _____

Do you practice tantra? (Y/N) _____

Do you practice sexual kung fu? (Y/N) _____

Spirituality

Do you believe? _____ In what? _____

Do you believe in God? _____ What kind? _____

Are you of any particular faith? _____ Which one? _____

Since? _____

Have you tried others? _____ Which ones? _____

Occupation

Occupation _____ Self-employed? (Y/N)

Hours of time spent working ___ Hours of time spent thinking about work ___

Amount of enjoyment achieved from work _____

Digestion

Estimated time of digestion from eating to movement? _____

Do you practice food combining? (Y/N) What kind? _____

Do you have flatulence? (Y/N)

What is the consistency of your stools? _____ What size? W_____ x L_____

How often do you have bowel movements? _____

What times of day? _____

How do your bowel movements smell? _____

Color of bowel movement? _____

Any undigested food matter? _____ What type? _____

What foods digest the best for you? _____

What foods could you digest better? _____

Are enemas a part of your practice? (Y/N)

Have you had colonic therapy? (Y/N)

How much do you have to exert yourself to sweat? _____

How does your sweat smell? _____

What is the color of your urine? _____

How often do you urinate? _____

How does your urine smell? _____

Do you practice urine therapy? (Y/N)

How does your food affect you energywise?_____

_____

_____

_____

_____

_____

Sleep

How many hours of sleep do you get per night? _____

What time do you go to sleep most often? _____

What time do you wake up most often? _____

Are you tired when you wake? (Y/N)

How close to bedtime do you eat? _____

Do you wake up during the night? (Y/N)

If yes, to do what?_____

What is your most memorable dream? _____

_____

_____

_____

_____

_____

Do you have nightmares? (Y/N)

Describe _____

_____

_____

_____

_____

Do you lucid dream? (Y/N)

Describe _____

_____

Do you wet your bed? (Y/N) How often?_____

Do you have wet dreams? (Y/N) How often?_____

Do you use an alarm clock? (Y/N) What time is it set to? _____

Do you sleep as long as you would like to?_____

Do you take naps during the day? _____ At what time? _____

What direction is your head pointing when you sleep? (N/S/E/W)

Are you warm when sleeping? (Y/N)

What is your bedding made of? _____

This part of the questionnaire helps us understand the psyche and motivations. Answer the questions quickly and in the order they appear. The more descriptive the better. It is often best to use the first things you think of, yet it all works.

Write the name of an animal and three words to describe it.

_____

Write the name of a second animal and three words to describe it.

_____

Write the name of a third animal and three words to describe it.

_____

You are walking along, and you find a path. It may be one you have seen before, one you have read about, or even one from fantasy. Please describe it.

What is it made of? _____

Where does it go? _____

What is the terrain? _____

What are the surroundings like? _____

List at least five adjectives describing the path. _____

_____

Next, your path leads you to find a book. Describe it. _____

_____

What is it made of?_____

What is its size? _____

What are its contents? _____

When was it made? _____

Who is the author, if any? _____

Then, you find your ideal cup. Describe it. _____

_____

What is it made of? _____

What does it contain, if anything? _____

What is its size? _____

What is its shape? _____

When was it made? _____

How or for what is it used? _____

List at least five adjectives describing the cup.

1._____

2._____

3._____

4._____

5._____

Finally, you encounter an impenetrable wall that extends in all directions (up, down, left, and right) into infinity as far as you can tell. What do you do?

_____

_____

_____

_____

_____

_____

_____

Recommended Reading

The Alchemist by Paolo Coelho

Be Your Own Doctor by Ann Wigmore

Complete Nutritional Food Facts by Sonia Newhouse

Composition and Facts About Foods by Ford Heritage

Conscious Eating by Gabriel Cousins

Diet for a New America by John Robbins

Enzyme Nutrition by Edward Howell

Fasting Can Save Your Life by Herbert Shelton

Fasting for Health by TC Fry

Hope for the Flowers by Trina Paulus

Illusions by Richard Bach

The Kin of Ata Are Waiting for You by Dorothy Bryant

Naturama by Ann Wigmore

The Raw Foods Resource Guide by Jeremy Safron

The Raw Truth by Jeremy Safron

Spiritual Nutrition and the Rainbow Diet by Gabriel Cousins

The Sprouting Book by Ann Wigmore

Survival into the 21st Century by Viktoras Kulvinskas

The Wheatgrass Book by Ann Wigmore

If you have a fast or type of cleanse that you would like to share, write us and let us know about it. If you have a great success story that you would love to share with people about fasting, send it to us, and we may print it in our next edition.

Loving Foods
P. O. Box 790358
Paia, HI 96779
www.lovingfoods.com

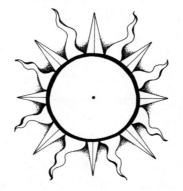

Glossary

Abundance: accepting the fact that there is always enough.

Albumen: the blood protein carrier manufactured in the stomach. High albumen levels are a sign of radiant good health, while albumen levels in the low twenties are indications of imminent death. Good internal hygiene and the occasional dry fast are excellent ways to raise albumen levels.

Assimilation: the ability to absorb nutrition.

Caloric value: how much energy a food will give.

Conception vessel: primary meridian going from the tongue to the perineum.

Elimination: the ability to excrete and remove.

Glycemic index: the glycolytic value of food; a list of sugar content.

Glycolytic rate: how fast sugar can be processed and stored by the liver and how much energy is received for work of digestion.

Governing vessel: primary meridian traveling the length of the spine from tailbone over the head onto the roof of the mouth.

Healing crisis: a time where our body feels challenged or could feel more excellent; the result of detoxification done too rapidly.

Living: bioactive containing the ability to sustain or create life.

Meridian/nadi: a pathway that rivers of energy travel through the body.

Organic water: water trapped in a living membrane or cell.

Raw: uncooked and unprocessed.

Sprout: the initial germination of a seed, nut, bean, or grain.

Toxin: an unwanted substance that has degenerating effects on the body.

Water: the stuff of life, H_2O.

Wheatgrass: a grass grown from hard wheat berries and a superpowerful source of chlorophyll and concentrated nutrition.

Raw Truth Catalog

The Raw Truth offers books, charts, and educational materials that support and enhance the raw food lifestyle.

Educational Materials

4 Living Food Group Chart, $10.00
A standard guideline for balanced raw food eating.

Exotic Fruit Chart, $15.00
A guide to uses, benefits, season availability, and more.

Fruit Chart, $10.00
Learn to identify and find out helpful facts about your favorite fruits.

The Raw Foods Resource Guide, $10.00
A great introduction to the basics of the raw food diet and lifestyle. Tons of information!

The Raw Truth, $20.00
Our most popular recipe book, filled with recipes and great information on tools and techniques.

Sprout Chart, $10.00
A great reference on how to sprout various beans, nuts, seeds, and grains.

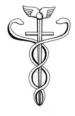

Loving Foods Merchandise

Clothing and Products

Sprout T-shirt (organic cotton or bamboo), $20.00

Sprout women's tank top (organic cotton), $20.00

Praktisac, $11.00
A fun toy that teaches you kung fu.

Spilanthia flowers, 4 for $1.00
Amazing mouth cleansers that are high in isobuterals
and Polynesian Eccinatia.

Geminations Herbal Color Bath, $7.00
Gem infused bath herbs for chakra balancing and vibrational medicine.

Geminations Herbal Teas, $5.00
Crystal charged herbal teas for enhanced living.

Fundi-Issemble CD, $18.00
Rastafarian drumming and chanting.

We also provide a wide range of food items, nutritional products, living food
culinary tools (juicers, dehydrators, blenders) and books by a variety of
authors on numerous subjects. E-mail us at allraw@lovingfoods.com for a
complete catalog. Please check our website, www.lovingfoods.com.

Loving Foods Retreats and Workshops

Experience all that life has to offer. Pick and eat exotic fruits right under the trees; learn creative and innovative new ways to prepare delicious raw food meals; practice yoga, chi kung, and kung fu; start and eat your own sprouts; learn how to identify wild foods; find out how to use food as medicine; and train your brain and maximize your potential. In other words, have the adventure of a lifetime. Come and relax, rejuvenate, and rejoice. We offer a variety of programs and a wide range of accommodations. We can provide for all dietary needs. We offer certification for teachers and chefs. Come and learn about yourself through the wonders of nature.

For more information, call (310) RAW-FOOD.

Group Workshops • Individual Retreats • Custom-Designed Training

Name _____ Age _____

Address _____

City _____ State _____ Zip _____

Phone # _____ Email _____

Interests:

❏ Fasting ❏ Chi kung ❏ Recipes ❏ Adventure

❏ Yoga ❏ Raw food ❏ Healing ❏ Cortical tissue maintenance

Times of year available _____

Location possibilities:
Hawaii, California, Oklahoma, New York, Florida, Vermont